HACKING LYME DISEASE

HACKING LYME DISEASE

A PRACTICAL GUIDE FOR
RECLAIMING YOUR HEALTH

CRISTINA RANDALL

HOUNDSTOOTH
PRESS

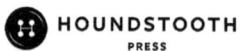

HACKING LYME DISEASE
A Practical Guide for Reclaiming Your Health

FIRST EDITION

ISBN   978-1-5445-3893-8   *Paperback*
         978-1-5445-3894-5   *Ebook*

This book is dedicated to anyone affected by Lyme Disease and coinfections, to those who have had to navigate a medical system that is still catching up and have had to demystify a myriad of changing symptoms. Maybe at one point they were called crazy or were told that it was all in their head. Many have shown such resilience and strength during their healing and were a huge source of information for my journey. I even learned to weigh their advice highly compared to accepted clinical practices. Many are so tired of an upward battle and just seek to be at peace with their body and find relief. They call them Lyme warriors for a reason. So this book is dedicated to you, Lyme warrior.

Lyme research is advancing in leaps and bounds. It is my hope that this book becomes largely outdated in the next decade and that the landscape for Lyme diagnosis and treatment completely changes.

CONTENTS

"Everyone has a doctor in him or her; we just have to help it in its work. The natural healing force within each one of us is the greatest force in getting well."

—HIPPOCRATES

INTRODUCTION

MY HEALTH DECLINE OVERNIGHT

Before I dive into the details of what I have learned about healing from Lyme Disease, I want to provide you with some context about my subjective experience with this disease and how my body was set up prior to developing symptoms. Also, this context is for you to get to know me better and view my experience with Lyme Disease in the backdrop of my history and decisions before getting sick. So let's dive right in and let me tell you more about myself.

From a young age, I've never been one to address emotional conflict head-on. I usually avoided any sort of conflict, within my family or friends, personal and professional relationships, wherever possible fleeing the situation. Over time, I let these inner conflicts with myself and with others accumulate. Each one added a weight that I carried with me and never let go of or dealt with, also never appreciating how the emotional and mental part of health can impact the physical. I also never came to terms with the conflict between my parents and how an abusive or conflictive environment growing up could have affected me as a child, or how the feelings from the disconnect I experienced with one of my parents stayed with me as I grew up.

As I learned later, a child up until the age of seven perceives conflict very differently than an adult, even if the emotional, mental, or physical abuse is not directed at the child. And even when the child is an observer, the child views it as a direct threat. One does not have to experience an explicitly traumatic event, such as a sudden death in the family, or a violent act for a trauma, however big or small, to impact one's health. Seemingly smaller traumatic or nontraumatic events can also take a toll.

Then as a child, I had the standard vaccines, without the knowledge of how they would affect my immune system or that other options existed. After I had braces as a teenager, a little steel wire was left to keep my teeth in place.

I had no idea that this supposedly benign wire would leech iron and nickel into my body for the next fifteen years. Over time, it would impair my immune system, increase my toxin burden, and later cause energetic imbalances in my body. I also learned later that a diet full of fat-soluble vitamins, such as K, D, and A as recommended by the Weston A. Price Foundation as being enough to build a strong jaw structure with healthy teeth, without needing additional support or intervention.

Before turning twenty-five, I had worked and traveled in more than thirty countries without any awareness about parasite prevention or treatment protocols. I had no idea that life's insults accumulate over time, such as the pathogens that were picked up, or the environmental toxins that we are exposed to, such as those when living in one of the most polluted cities in the world for a decade. I was brought up in the backdrop of Western conventional medicine where antibiotics were given out to fix urinary tract infections and birth control pills were presented as the main option to regulate hormones.

Oral birth control I learned later in life has many negative, downstream health effects that were never communicated to me when I started taking it.

Also, when living in a state of constant stress in my professional endeavors, I thought it was OK to go days without having a bowel movement or skipping a day.

I now realize how important it is to have a daily, healthy bowel movement, otherwise toxins build up and are recirculated throughout your body.

I grew up wanting to take on the world and not accepting no for an answer, chasing achievements, graduating top of my class, and earning a level of success by hard work in entrepreneurship, not paying attention to any emotional or spiritual collateral damage along the way. I left expressions of creativity and art for engineering. I prioritized hard work over fun and enjoyment. I practiced only one form of movement and that was to push myself to the extreme. In competitive sports, I physically exhausted my body without recovering, flying across the world for a few days just to run a marathon, for example.

I didn't have a spiritual practice, and I didn't set many limitations. I hadn't yet realized that energy is a finite, precious resource. I had a network of friends but not a sense of community I wanted to build. Both professionally and personally, I was dissatisfied with how my life wasn't aligned fully with my core values and the vision of how I wanted to serve in the world. The late-night work sessions, the stress, sugar, alcohol, skipped meals, the unprocessed emotional trauma—all this sacrifice seemed part of getting to the next big thing, chasing after that next deal.

Fast forward to my early thirties when I had an infected wisdom tooth taken out by a conventional dentist. I found this strange because my other wisdom teeth that were extracted never caused problems. Months later, the neighboring tooth developed a cavitation, and I opted for a root canal because that appeared to be the only option at the time. I took prescribed antibiotics and thought the problem had gone away. The conventional dentist deemed the procedure a "success."

Later, I learned that conventional dentists don't fully clean these sites and leave in the periodontal ligament, which becomes a breeding ground and reservoir for bad bacteria. Root canals are a point of controversy and are not always the best option. It is impossible to fully clean a root canal tooth, despite what conventional dentists claim, and the site will become a source of latent infection, which your body will always deal with afterward. The decision to get a root canal should be carefully evaluated with a biological dentist. Many progressive practitioners and biological dentists recommend leaving the root canal only for a few years as a temporary solution. If an illness like a cancer arises later in life, the root canal should likely be removed.

Around about the same time, I went on a camping trip in California, a region endemic with ticks with zero awareness of Lyme Disease and the recommended protective measures for preventing insect bites. I brought my dog, mopping up all things on the forest floor and afterward slept in my tent.

I didn't feel a tick bite or see a bull's-eye rash. Immediately after the trip, I didn't feel different or become symptomatic. It was only months later, after I came back from a trip across the world where I was to speak to hundreds of people, including heads of governments when I was sleep deprived, dehydrated, confused by time zones, and poorly nourished that I began to experience symptoms. I caught a stomach bug upon return and my health then went downhill. It was like nothing I had ever experienced and hit me like a giant wave in the face. Lyme brought me to my knees. For several months, my body progressively stopped responding. Sometimes I lost vision or feeling in one side of my body, had heart palpitations, panic attacks, forgot names, or couldn't think clearly, couldn't sleep for days, couldn't breathe, had dizziness, light-headedness, faintness, pain, had a bedridden fatigue and weakness, and I experienced a suffering physically, mentally, and spiritually like I had never known. I took antibiotics which only seemed to make it worse.

What followed in the next several months can only be described as a wild goose chase across three countries and more than forty doctors, dozens of ER visits, and hundreds of thousands of dollars in out-of-pocket medical expenses. It was the scariest time of my life, with so much uncertainty. Now in hindsight, I realize how fortunate I was that within five months of developing symptoms, a determined naturopath ran a specialty Lyme panel and everything became clear.

HOW TO USE THIS BOOK

Once the Lyme and coinfections diagnosis became clear, I started a journey to understand what these infections were, how they affected my body, and how I could get better. What I learned and the content that follows in this book was not readily available in the conventional or alternative medical system. In fact, it took me much time to navigate and organize the myriad of information with the help of experts and specialist practitioners and guided by my own self-experimentation. The content that follows is a brain download of the knowledge I accumulated in the years after my diagnosis. It is my intention to share the lessons learned through my own mistakes and hardships so that the reader's healing journey is smoother.

Information around Lyme is confusing and overwhelming to say the least. So the intention of this book is to help you through this learning curve and provide additional clarity during your recovery journey.

Read this book as a guide. Take notes, highlight passages, check out the resources and links. The information is the result of hundreds of conversations with experts—MDs, immunologists, naturopaths, neurologists, healers, nurse practitioners, biohackers, and other people with Lyme—and knowledge from courses, observations, firsthand experimentation with various herbs and pharmaceuticals, and hands-on learning with the motivation and hunger that my life depended on it.

Please use this as a practical resource, meant to assist your learning curve. Specific practitioners, stories, products, and services have been carefully selected. The content that follows is essentially what I would've loved to know during my recovery. Some of the most valuable and useful information tends to be from people actually undergoing treatment and recovering themselves. Every person is different. There is no single, right formula, but you may encounter tips or gems of information that might help you turn a corner. I've done my best to compile the gems that other people have shared with me.

It is meant to be concise and unfiltered so you can focus your energy on healing and get back to your life. The amount of information out there can be overwhelming, so the aim of this book is to summarize and do some of the work for you. This book was also written during the height of the COVID-19 pandemic where we had to be self-sufficient, pursue detox practices and therapies at home, and minimize trips to clinics or medical facilities. I've realized that our bodies are a pharmacy, capable of producing all sorts of biochemicals, which can lead to our own healing.

I wrote this also to support informed consent, which is the concept of the patient being fully informed and empowered to make decisions in the best interest of his or her health. If everyone had an infinite budget for health, healing from Lyme would be easier. Unfortunately, the path to wellness can be expensive. So another aim of this book is to make information, normally hidden behind costly specialist consultations along with trial and error and out-of-pocket expenses, more readily available to you. When doing my own research, I never came across a single resource like this book that brought together the information and curated content for impact and usefulness. Lyme and other coinfections are so confusing and complex for both practitioners and patients. To make matters worse, one is also caught in the middle of the politics associated with the disease and feels abandoned by a conventional medical system. The scope of this book does not include the politics and history around Lyme Disease, but readers are encouraged to refer to other excellent resources on the topic (Raxlen 2019; Newby 2020). Hopefully, this book serves as a compass to orient yourself and to understand the current options available for healing.

WHY YOU CAN TRUST ME

First a disclaimer: I am not a doctor, and I don't have medical training. I wrote what follows based on my own personal health journey and investigation to heal myself. Not being a medical professional or practitioner, nothing I do is contingent on the content of the material here or the success of this publication. I also have no interests or affiliations with the products listed. I have nothing to hide and nothing to benefit from publishing this. I'm not concerned about losing any licenses. I've already gone through the learning curve associated with Lyme Disease and made my share of mistakes. I actually started this book as a reference for myself and a way of keeping notes. Now my primary interest is to share what I've learned from my own healing journey so that fewer people have to suffer. As I tackled my own healing, I became more aware of the historical context of our perceptions and biases in medical practices today. So I did my best to set these predominant perceptions aside and home in on the scientific data and on what really works, by my own account and by the recommendations of others who recovered.

I come from an engineering background and approached my own healing as any other problem. I had a maniacal desire to get better and to do whatever it took to get my life back. I tried practically everything I've described in this book, from the therapies to the detox protocols. I threw everything at the problem and tried countless things until I got better. I didn't stop until I got my quality of life back and returned to my "baseline." Since there is no single, clear path to recovery when healing from Lyme, hundreds of therapies will also compete for your attention. Managing everything might seem like a full-time job; at least it was a full-time job for me during a period of my life. This book is meant to take some complexity out of the process.

HEALING MENTALITY AND PRACTITIONERS

You have likely gotten here after navigating a complex medical system and have learned to trust your intuition. You probably know already how frustrating the process can be and that many conventional MDs do not recognize chronic Lyme. Maybe you have a binder of test results after seeing many doctors, have received many different diagnoses, and tried to make sense of a changing set of confusing symptoms.

Throughout the rest of the treatment, you will still need to trust your intuition. Yet you still need to work with a Lyme specialist who has experience in diagnosing and treating the Lyme condition. You will also likely work with other specialists, such as a cardiologist and a neurologist to eliminate other possibilities and also to review affected organs in coordination with your Lyme doctor. You will ultimately be a champion or advocate for your own health all the time, but working with a specialist is indispensable. If you don't know of any specialists in your area, look at the International Lyme and Associated Diseases Society (ILADS) directory www.ilads.org and find a Lyme-literate doctor (LLMD). You need to work with an LLMD as you will be spinning your wheels with a conventional MD who is not trained or well versed in Lyme. For most MDs who are not Lyme literate, talking about the topic seems taboo. You should find an experienced LLMD as the priority, since the dosing of any protocol or the order of different treatments can mark the difference of success.

Aside from an LLMD and additional specialists, try to seek guidance from a generalist holistic practitioner to put things into perspective and adjust priorities during treatment. For example, when you speak to a specialist, they will narrowly focus on their field; a Lyme expert will want to kill the Lyme, a mold expert will want to prioritize mold, and so on. So sometimes it's easy to go down rabbit roles and forget to assess your body's priorities and imbalances.

Chronic illnesses like Lyme Disease are difficult to treat, and you may encounter many practitioners along your journey to health. Be conscious of giving power to white coats or, in the case of alternative medicine, well-intentioned healers or holistic practitioners. In a study at the Mayo Clinic in 2017, medical records of more than 200 patients who came for a second opinion, 20 percent of these opinions were a totally different diagnosis than the original diagnosis, and 88 percent of the time the second opinion differed substantially (Van Such et al. 2017). In other words, expert opinion can differ so significantly that you should take ownership of the decision making. Using a business analogy, one should become the CEO of one's own health.

Another important role that often goes unnoticed or underappreciated throughout the healing journey is the "go-to" person who provides support and helps navigate through the myriad of decisions that need to be made. This person may be a spouse, family member, or close friend, and sometimes they are listed as the emergency contact. They should have a deep firsthand understanding of your situation, will look out for your best interests, and step in when you are not able to make a decision.

You will also have to experiment to a certain degree on yourself, since each body reacts differently to medications and treatments. Have patience. There is no overnight fix, although the tips listed here are meant to accelerate your healing, and the process will take time. Starting "low and slow" is the recommended approach always; also, trying one change at a time as it will be easier to track which changes are having an impact. Practitioners can give you their opinions, which may be varied. Doctors can be wrong. And the whole treatment process can be confusing, but ultimately, it comes down to your decision. Sometimes in the current wild, wild, west world of Lyme treatment, we need this reminder.

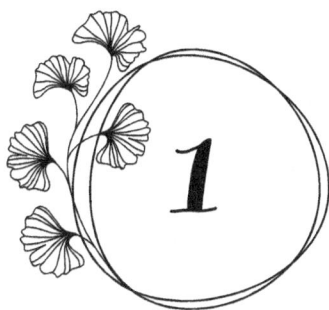

1

OVERVIEW

WHAT IS LYME?

Ticks have been around for hundreds of thousands of years. In one study, researchers did genomic sequencing on the 146 genomes of *Borrelia burgdorferi* and found that its most recent ancestor is more than 60,000 years old (Walter et al. 2017). Indeed, humans have been living with Lyme for a long time. Genetic analysis discovered Lyme Disease in a 5,300-year-old ice mummy in the eastern Alps (Sonenshine and Macaluso 2017).

The disease was named after the town Lyme, Connecticut where in the '70s clusters of children in the same areas around the same time started developing joint pain, rashes, and fevers, which were thought to be juvenile arthritis. Several years later, Dr. Alan Steere identified the disease as being transmitted from ticks. Then in 1982, William Burgdorfer, a medical entomologist, identified the spirochete, a spiral-shaped bacteria, as being the causative agent of the disease, and so *Borrelia burgdorferi* received its name.

Lyme today is eight times more prevalent than HIV and three times more prevalent than breast cancer (Lyme Policy Wonk 2019). The Centers for Disease Control and Prevention (CDC) reports 470,000 in the United States alone per year, which is more than cases of breast cancer, HIV, and hepatitis C combined, yet experts believe this number doesn't come close to reality, since only those who reported a tick bite within six weeks of a positive Western blot are factored into this number ("Data and Surveillance" 2022). A recent study based on commercial insurance claim data suggests actual cases are most likely underreported and generate over $1 billion in medical costs (Hook et al. 2022). Today, it is the most common and fastest-growing vector-borne disease in the United States and Europe, according to the CDC ("Lyme Disease" 2022). It is estimated that in the northeast United States, up to half of the ticks can carry *Borrelia*, the causative agent of Lyme Disease. Whereas in areas of California, it is estimated at a lower percentage, such as 5 percent of the ticks. Today, cases of Lyme Disease are turning up in areas that had never been thought to be endemic, with speculation around global warming being a driving factor in its spread, along with deforestation, urbanization, hunting, and the increased deer population (Pfeiffer 2018). Indeed, researchers predict that climate change, loss of biodiversity, and population growth will accelerate the spread of many zoonotic diseases like Lyme ("Drivers of Zoonotic Diseases" 2019).

Lyme is a controversial illness because it is so difficult to diagnose and culture. In other words, when you take the blood from an infected human or animal, you cannot easily grow it, which means we can't tell who has it and who doesn't. Also, there are more than 300 strains that are not detected by the standard test called ELISA.

The two-pronged testing approach currently in use was never developed considering the case of chronic Lyme.

Lyme is also difficult to detect because in most cases, people do not remember a tick bite or never had a bull's-eye rash (which in many cases is caused by a tick no larger than the size of this dot: .). The expression of the rash, otherwise known as erythema migrans, can also vary, with some rashes showing the telltale concentric rings or bull's-eye and others smaller, less obvious. In fact, very rarely does it appear as the typical telltale bull's-eye. To many who have not seen a tick or rash, a Lyme diagnosis may come across as surprising.

The comparison below gives a sense of how small in size ticks are and why they are difficult to spot.

Before the tick bites you, it uses chemicals that act like an anesthetic so you don't feel the tick bite. Also, as you can see, the nymph-stage tick is the most difficult to identify. The ticks are so small, almost indistinguishable from specs of dirt, and they're too small to feel them crawling on you. Although ticks do not have good vision or hearing, their sense of smell is heightened. They can detect carbon dioxide and lactic acid emissions and also odors from microbial colonies on a person's skin. Ticks do not prefer sunlight, opting for locations not readily seen, such as in hair or under clothes. The time it takes to transmit an infection is a hotly debated topic. Some doctors

WESTERN BLACKLEGGED TICK

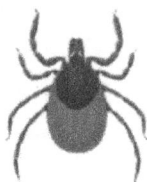

Adult female 2.5 mm

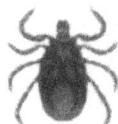

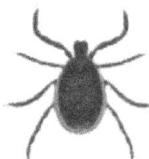

Adult male 2.0mm

Nymph 1.0 mm

Larva 0.5 mm

EASTERN BLACKLEGGED TICK

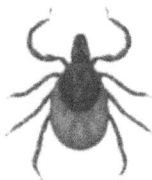

Adult female 2.5 mm

Adult male 2.0mm

Nymph 1.0 mm

Larva 0.5 mm

SIZE COMPARISON

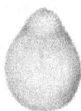

Sesame seed 3.0 mm

Poppy seed 1.0 mm

claim that if the tick was not attached for at least twenty-four to forty-eight hours, they have nothing to worry about. This is not true as there is enough research to show that infection can be spread in an even short amount of time, even within several minutes of being attached. Lyme is also transmitted through mosquitoes, mites, fleas, biting flies, via sex, from mother to child, and survives blood banks (Middelveen et al. 2014). Household pets can also be a source of infection. If you have a cat, it may have transferred *Bartonella* to you. If you have a dog, you may have gotten Lyme from the fleas.

Lyme is a systemic illness that affects multiple organs. Within days of being infected, Lyme spreads throughout your body. The spirochete's corkscrew-like shape and tail, called a flagellum, allow it to quickly travel through dense tissues in the body, through organs, across the blood-brain barrier, outrunning the immune cells, and create a range of symptoms. It then becomes a burden on the immune system and may worsen other health conditions or be accompanied by nutrient deficiency, heavy-metal toxicity, mold mycotoxin, adrenal dysfunction, parasites, GI issues, and candida.

Lyme Disease is often called the great imitator and is frequently misdiagnosed as multiple sclerosis, Bell's palsy, bipolar disorder, schizophrenia, arthritis, depression, optic neuritis, meningitis, nerve damage, Ménière's syndrome, chronic fevers, strange ticks in the ear, random soreness, brain fog, and the list goes on and on (Stricker and Fesler 2018). Indeed, it is thought to be behind many physiological and neurological illnesses ("Drivers of Zoonotic Diseases" 2019).

An observational crowdsourced project called MyLymeData.org

which records data of more 14,000 people with Lyme Disease, found that 72 percent of the respondents were misdiagnosed before obtaining a Lyme diagnosis. The most common misdiagnoses include fibromyalgia (43 percent), chronic fatigue (43 percent), thyroid disorder (26 percent), and rheumatoid arthritis (17 percent), progressive neurologic conditions, such as multiple sclerosis (12 percent), as well as Parkinson's Disease and ALS (5 percent) (Johnson 2019). People can be on a spectrum from being mildly symptomatic to being in a wheelchair and in a critical state with major damage to organs.

Research has found that Lyme Disease creates inflammation markers that specifically target nerve cells called glial cells, which are responsible for regeneration. While the immune system targets pathogens, tissues are damaged, and as a result, permanent damage can occur over many years and multiple bites (Ramesh et al. 2013). In fact, many of the leading Lyme practitioners comment that their patients who suffer from Alzheimer's, Parkinson's, ALS, and multiple sclerosis commonly test positive for *Borrelia B*. In multiple studies, Lyme has also been found in tissue samples from multiple sclerosis patients (Marshall 1988). Indeed, many practitioners believe that Lyme Disease and, if not caught and treated, tick-borne illnesses more generally may indeed be a catalyst for chronic or autoimmune illnesses, which are estimated to affect 50 million Americans (Phillips and Parish 2020).

THE BODY WITH LYME

The strain of Lyme or other tick-borne diseases a tick carries will depend on the species of the tick and its geographic location. Certain strains of *Borrelia* are more likely to present with neuromuscular symptoms, whereas others have a relapsing fever as a symptom.

People with untreated or undertreated Lyme can experience hundreds of symptoms and can be affected by chemical sensitivities, flare-ups during a menstrual cycle, unexpected allergies, bruising, intolerance to alcohol, heightened sensitivity to insect bites, increased time needed for recovery, and strange, unexplainable symptoms or sensations. People affected feel like their body is failing in multiple different and confusing ways. Lyme can mimic many other things, such as mold illness. However, the one distinguishing symptom only found with Lyme is a wandering or "migrating" sensation of symptoms, such as arthralgias or pain. Spirochetes have an affinity for areas in the body with low blood flow and high in fat or sugar, such as connective tissues, joints, synovial fluid, nerve tissues, and the brain. The ability of the spirochete to travel so well explains why these symptoms can migrate from different parts of the body. Symptoms are found in multiple areas of a person's body with complaints of musculoskeletal pain, neurological symptoms, endocrine imbalances, cardiorespiratory, and gastrointestinal disturbances.

TYPES OF LYME AND COINFECTIONS

Ninety percent of people infected with *Borrelia* may also be harboring coinfections, which are acquired at the time of the tick bite. Studies show that at least 60 percent of people with Lyme are diagnosed with one or more coinfection (Johnson 2019). Indeed, it is believed that a tick can spread more than 200 different types of bacteria and many types of viruses, which means that many chronic Lyme patients might be infected with many different types of microbes at the same time (Zhang et al. 2014).

Many symptoms, such as clouded thinking, interrupted sleep, low energy, and so forth are a result of overproduction of cytokines. Cytokines are produced by white blood cells to fight the infection, but when we produce too much, the result is the symptoms that we experience. In fact, other nonrelated Lyme conditions, such as yeast overgrowth and mold toxicity can generate cytokines that look like Lyme symptoms. The most intense symptoms will be different for different people as Lyme is believed to attack the weakest area of your body.

Hundreds of symptoms may be attributed to *Borrelia* and many more to coinfections. Here is a list of typical symptoms attributed to each microbe:

BORRELIA	BARTONELLA	BABESIA
Flu-like symptoms	Constant anxiety	Brain fog/cognitive impairment
Swollen lymph nodes	Unusual neurological symptoms	Drenching night/day sweats or fevers/chills
Fevers	Anxiety, anger, irritability, panic attacks	Palpitations (POTS)
Stiff neck	Eye pain, visual disturbances, conjunctivitis	Air hunger or shortness of breath
Wandering or "migrating" arthralgias	Skin: "Tracks"/striae (red/purple stretch marks) that do not follow skin planes	Costal pain
Headache on back of the head	Temporal headache	Frontal headache

BORRELIA	BARTONELLA	BABESIA
Fatigue/poor stamina	Bone pain on hips, soles of feet, and small joints	Adrenal fatigue/ orthostatic hypertension
Myalgias	Lymphadenopathy— lumps and bumps. Swollen lymph nodes	Dizziness, loss of balance
	Day sweats	Acute anxiety, panic attacks
	Abdominal pain, bowel issues	Nausea, anemia
	Electrical shock sensations	Numbness and tingling/ burning pain
	Seizures/encephalopathy	Cyclical, worsening of symptoms every three to four weeks
	Unusual rashes	Enlarged spleen, easy bruising

In addition to these three microbes, other Lyme viruses, anaplasmosis, ehrlichia, chlamydia pneumoniae, which are part of the tick bite and other viruses, such as Epstein Barr Virus (EBV), Cytomegalovirus (CMV), and Human Herpesvirus 6 (HHV6), which normally are dominant but activated when the immune system is overburdened can cause a variety of other symptoms. Indeed, the variety of microbes that each individual may be dealing with when they are infected is extremely varied and can make treatment even more challenging, especially when these individual infections are not properly identified.

In an article in the *Proceedings of the National Academy of Sciences (PNAS)*, it is estimated that 99 percent of microbes have yet to be discovered, which is a humbling thought that many potentially pathogenic vector-borne microbes have yet to be identified and understood (Locey and Lennon 2016).

WHERE IS IT?

Lyme Disease has been documented in every state in the United States and in many countries around the world. It's showing up in places where communities and local doctors are unfamiliar with the disease. With the suburban sprawl, more people are living in deer-inhabited areas. Some areas are even overpopulated with deer or other carriers, such as the white-footed mouse, because of an imbalance of predator and prey in the ecosystem. Also, ticks are not killed off in the winter with the warmer seasons and with a warmer climate. Lyme has actually been described as the first epidemic of climate change (Pfeiffer 2018). Although many associate Lyme Disease with ticks, various other vectors can carry Lyme and coinfections. Many other savvy practitioners recognize the rising prevalence of other carriers, such as black flies and mosquitoes. A mosquito, for example, can transmit Lyme and coinfections to a human, after it has bit an infected animal.

The number of confirmed and probable Lyme Disease cases in the United States more than doubled from 2001 to 2015, as can be seen from this map from the CDC (Centers for Disease Control and Prevention 2021).

MAPS OF LYME DISEASE CASES

2001

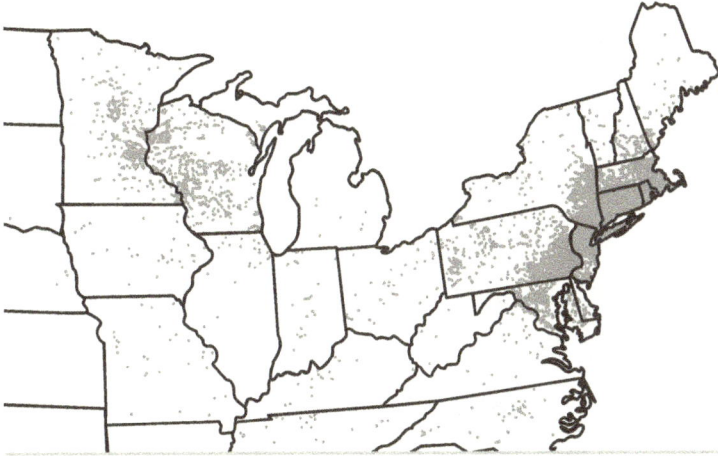

2015

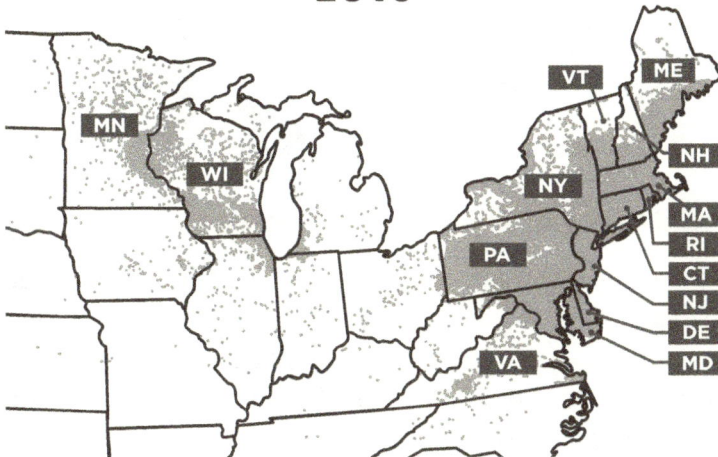

Map Credit: Annotation by Katie Park/NPR. Source of data: https://www.cdc.gov/lyme/stats/index.html

RESEARCH

Much of the current situation around Lyme Disease can be understood within the context of the research dedicated to the disease.

NIH FUNDING FOR RESEARCH
($ Millions)

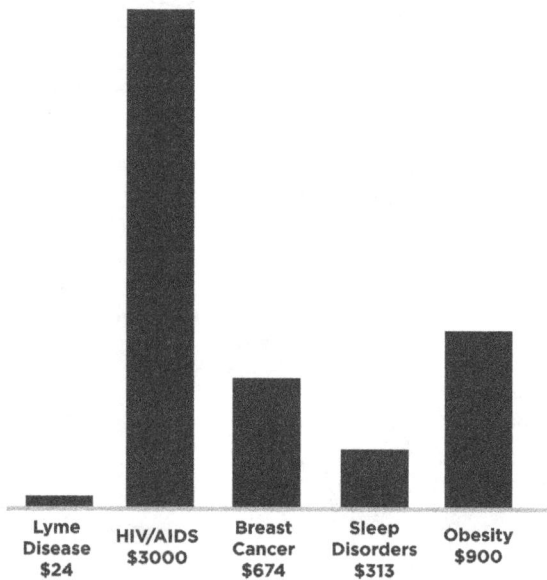

Lyme Disease $24	HIV/AIDS $3000	Breast Cancer $674	Sleep Disorders $313	Obesity $900

The National Institutes of Health (NIH) has funded the greatest amount of vector-borne disease studies. However, this amount pales in comparison to other categories. For perspective, Lyme Disease receives 0.2 percent of the public funding that HIV/AIDS does ("Federal Funding of Tick-Borne Diseases" 2011). Indeed, there are only three NIH-funded randomized controlled trials over the last twenty years, as the following figure shows the number of clinical trials for Lyme Disease in comparison to other categories.

NUMBER OF CLINICAL TRIALS IN INFECTIOUS DISEASES

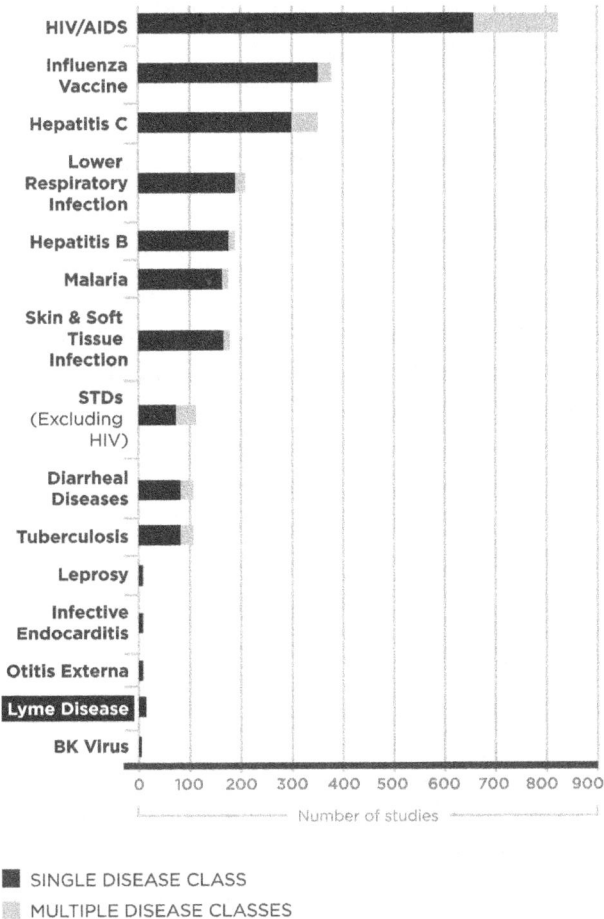

From Goswami et al., "The State of Infectious Diseases Clinical Trials: A Systematic Review of clinicaltrials.gov," *PLoS One* 8, no. 10 (October 2016): e77086, https://doi.org/10.1371/journal.pone.0077086.

Unfortunately, there are many studies that show certain herbal antibiotics work in a petri dish, such as grape-seed extract or essential oils, but we have no evidence to say that they work in humans. Efficacy in vitro does not translate to efficacy in vivo. To date, there are few human studies in terms of which antibiotics or combinations of antibiotics work for certain infections. As a result, treatment is guided by clinical experience and depends on the skill of the practitioner.

At the time of writing, the scientific community has developed multiple vaccines for COVID-19 in parallel in record time and responded in a way that we have never seen. As a global scientific community, we are capable of going from a viral genome sequence to a vaccine in a number of days, which is astonishing. However, for Lyme Disease, multiple attempts have been made for better therapeutics and diagnostic tools, a failed vaccine tried, yet people every day are still suffering from this debilitating disease. Other conditions such as autoimmune conditions and certain types of cancer are light-years ahead compared to where we are with Lyme. However, as public awareness increases, private funding and groups like the Global Lyme Alliance and the Bay Area Lyme Foundation are emerging and starting to make headway.

PREVENTION

Lyme Disease is now endemic in many areas and has been discovered in areas not suspected to ever have Lyme. Also, the immune system does not retain a memory of Lyme Disease like it does with other infections to clear it more efficiently the next time we encounter it. Rather, you can get Lyme Disease multiple times with each new tick bite. So awareness and prevention are key.

The book *Preventing Lyme & Other Tick-Borne Diseases* by Alexis Chesney reviews at length different strategies around preventing tick bites, even describing "tick traps" that discourage tick presence around your property (2020). For example, some practical measures that you can take within your yard include removing leaf piles and wood piles, moving equipment and playsets out of shaded areas, promoting landscaping that encourages light and minimizing shaded areas, reducing shrubs that attract deer and other wildlife, as well as taking measures to reduce pests around the property. For other natural tick-control measures, chickens or hens which feed on ticks can also reduce tick population. Keep the grass cut short and also place a three-foot perimeter of wood chips or gravel between your yard and any tall grasses or wooded areas. Ticks don't like crossing these areas as they are hot and dry. Around the home, another major risk factor are pets. Sleeping with pets is not advisable and frequent tick checks are recommended. Some pet stores carry natural herbal products (for example, a product called PetzLife Tickz) that the pet ingests every day in their food, which helps repel ticks so they do not attach. Permethrin, an insecticide that acts as a neurotoxin for insects, has been identified as being the most effective repellent. It is a man-made contact insecticide, similar to a naturally occurring chemical derived from the dried flowers of the chrysanthemum.

It has been used by the army to protect soldiers and livestock for years. You can also buy insect repellent clothing with permethrin, and there are several companies that treat clothes with permethrin, such as Insect Shield. Ticks typically can reach you around your feet, so pants, socks, and shoes treated with permethrin are useful, along with hats or head coverings in case they fall from trees. Although permethrin is an excellent option on clothes, it is not recommended on skin for extended periods. So soaking yourself in permethrin for life is not a wise option as it affects the central nervous system, even though it might be justified for short trips in high-risk areas. For direct application on the skin, there are several options reviewed by Consumer Reports which publishes detailed ratings, also available on their website. It is worth mentioning that each of the top-ranked products in a Consumer Reports study published in 2016 have DEET. For those who opt to use a more natural, less-toxic alternative, a company called Cedarcide offers a versatile spray containing cedarwood oil.

Unfortunately, no major clinical or conclusive studies have been done that objectively rank bug spray alternatives. Depending on which practitioner you ask, many will recommend different options. For example, many practitioners recommend Solvarome essential oil, which is a combination of lavender, rosemary, thyme oil, cypress, and rose geranium. To determine what really works, you will need to test sprays and strategies and be the guinea pig; try different things and observe which are more effective at preventing bites. The strategy will also differ depending on the insect of concern. For mosquitoes, citronella and lemongrass can be effective, whereas for ticks, geranium is better. You can also experiment by incorporating more garlic, onions, and grapefruit into your diet and by decreasing your sweets.

For taking internally to prevent tick bites, although there are no randomized controlled studies in humans, in animal studies, *Cistus incanus* when taken internally as a tea has been incredibly effective in repelling ticks. Many recommend drinking up to three or four cups of *Cistus incanus* per day for protection against tick bites. Another approach to prevention is by prophylactically taking different herbal combinations. Stephen Buhner in his book *Healing Lyme* recommends the herb astragalus (worth mentioning here that it may be contraindicated for long-term use in people with autoimmune conditions or autoimmune tendencies or predisposition to autoimmunity) (Buhner 2015). Other practitioners may recommend combinations of herbs, such as andrographis, cryptolepis, skutterleria, and Japanese knotweed to mention a few. Also, there are combination tinctures, such as the cocktail sold by Biopure that can be helpful. This book does not dive into dosing recommendations or provide guidance on treatment. The reader is encouraged to work with a Lyme-literate doctor for specific treatment protocols.

RECENT TICK BITE

You are likely not reading this due to an acute infection or tick bite. Nonetheless, if you were bitten by a tick, you should start treatment right away. Some doctors will recommend a wait-and-see approach; however, given what is at stake and the potential for chronic infection with a more extended treatment course, it is recommended to treat for *at least five to six weeks* with a tetracycline antibiotic or ideally an antibiotic combination to cover multiple coinfections. Unfortunately, the typical treatment of doxycycline as recommended by the CDC has been proven to be ineffective (Cameron et al. 2014). Due to the lower efficacy with the standard course of doxycycline, ILADS recommends continuous treatment until symptoms resolve. Many practitioners will also cover the coinfection's *Babesia* and *Bartonella*, using herbs like cryptolepis and sida acuta.

If you are not able to get the right care and attention, search immediately for a local LLMD in your area through the ILADS directory. Erythema migraines have become a hallmark symptom used to determine if the bite is infectious, but this sign is not reliable as many people develop Lyme Disease without ever having a red rash at the site. Also, if you see the tick on you, there is a special way to remove it as follows:

- Use a pair of fine-tipped tweezers with pointed ends or better yet, tweezers specifically designed for tick removal.
- Grasp the tick as close to the skin's surface as possible and pull upward with steady pressure. Do not twist or jerk the tick, as that could leave its head or other parts still in the skin.
- Do not burn it, squeeze it, or apply any substances to it, as the tick might regurgitate more infection through the skin, worsening the situation.
- Send the tick off for testing as this analysis will confirm any infections and help inform treatment, if necessary.

Opinions are mixed as to what to topically apply in the area. Some practitioners recommend iodine; others recommend different homeopathic remedies.

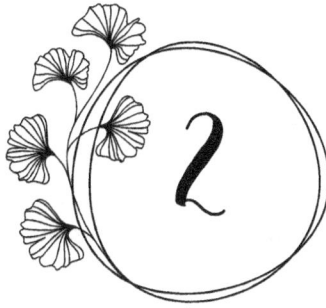

2

TESTING

According to the CDC, Lyme Disease is a clinical diagnosis based on signs and symptoms, and testing is helpful if used correctly as a secondary aid (Centers for Disease Control and Prevention 2022). In terms of testing, the topic is controversial, since it is recognized by patients and practitioners alike that the standard, most readily available two-tiered approach is not reliable. A study conducted a meta-analysis of eight scientific articles and determined the sensitivity of this test to be 46 percent (Stricker and Johnson 2010).

As part of the two-tiered approach, the enzyme-linked immunosorbent assay or ELISA is first used. Then if the ELISA is positive, the Western blot test which has higher specificity is then run. Unfortunately, there are multiple issues with this approach:

- The Western blot test was developed by matching antibodies in the human blood with a single strain of *Borrelia* from

Europe, ignoring the full range of proteins expressed by the hundreds of strains of *Borrelia* reported in the United States and worldwide including relapsing fever *Borrelia*. On top of using only one strain of the many antibodies expressed, just ten were deemed diagnostic. Even Immunetics, the company that manufactures the Western blot and sells it to LabCorp, has found that the alternative Western blot banding patterns produce better results for Lyme Disease patients.

- Both the ELISA and Western blot use "indirect testing" which looks at the immune cells produced, not the pathogen itself. Both IgM and IgG immunoglobulins are produced in response to the infection and are classified by their weight. The CDC considers a test positive if two out of three IgM bands are positive or if five out of ten IgG bands are positive. However, it can take a few weeks for the body to produce an immune response that is detectable, so these tests are unable to immediately tell whether someone is infected. This can be problematic, since patients have the best chance of a "clean" or uncomplicated recovery if treatment starts early. Also, these tests assume that the patient's immune system can mount a response to generate titers, a measure of the number of antibodies in the blood, which isn't always the case.

- The problem with blood testing is that the Lyme bacteria is not always in the blood; it can hide in synovial fluid or tissues. A blood test is a snapshot of a moment in time and does not represent what is going on in the whole body or in the other places where Lyme can be more concentrated.

After receiving a negative Lyme test, many people accept the results at face value and end up mistakenly receiving other diagnoses, such as adrenal fatigue, chronic EBV, or Hashimoto. Regardless of the test results, it is important to understand your symptom picture. For example, there is a questionnaire called the Horowitz score that calculates the probability of you having Lyme based on symptoms alone. If your tests are negative and you believe that you might have Lyme, even just by symptoms or the Horowitz score, make an appointment with a nearby LLMD as soon as possible.

Remember, Lyme is a clinical diagnosis and the standard two-tiered approach is not reliable. Unfortunately, a clinical diagnosis depends on the knowledge, training, and experience of the doctor. In many areas of the world with the exception of the northeast and north-central portions of the United States, many doctors are not specifically trained to recognize or treat Lyme and coinfections. Many doctors without experience in Lyme Disease may even treat the topic as taboo.

SPECIALIZED LABS

The following tests are specific to Lyme and offered by specialty labs. Unfortunately, these are not normally covered by insurance and are only ordered through LLMDs or practitioners who treat Lyme Disease.

TEST	TEST RESOURCES
Lyme Antibody (Indirect)	Unlike the two-tiered ELISA test, Igenex uses more than one strain of bacteria as the basis of their test. They are the only laboratory that uses a human-derived strain as opposed to a tick-derived strain. It is an indirect test that relies on the immune response. Since these antibodies can linger even when the infection is gone, results can indicate exposure at some point in the past but do not confirm that an infection is active. Full Igenex panels can be expensive, and some patients opt for the Tick Plex by Armin labs as a more general filter.
Cytokine Panel	This panel is offered by a lab in Germany called Armin Labs. A cytokine panel is useful as it provides insight into inflammation, but a knowledgeable practitioner is needed for its interpretation.
Elispot	By Armin Labs, the Elispot uses T cells which are immune cells that help the body fight off infection and have a memory of around six weeks. Although it does not necessarily indicate an active infection, it will test positive if your immune system has been active against Lyme or other microbes in the last six weeks.
DNA Connections	At the time of writing, DNA Connections is one of the few labs that offers direct-to-consumer at-home labs. They also offer analysis of teeth that are extracted. DNA Connections offer urine tests which can be helpful after provoking the microbes through exercise or red light. One of the downsides of DNA testing is that it does not effectively distinguish between living and dead organisms.
Tick Testing	Tick Report, Igenex, and Ticknology all offer tick testing.
PCR (Direct Testing)	The PCR is a direct test for the presence of the germ. These tests have high specificity meaning that if you test positive, you definitely have it. Unfortunately, since the microbes may not be in the blood or caught in the sample, a positive PCR is unlikely. An enhanced version of the PCR called the Fish increases the chances of finding the microbe. There is also a specialized version to detect *Bartonella* offered by Galaxy Diagnostics Labs where the growth of *Bartonella* is enhanced on special growing media before the PCR test is performed, which increases the chance of detection. Insurance also commonly does not offer coverage unless PCR is positive. A PCR can also be taken from other samples, such as cerebral spinal fluid or even from the umbilical cord.

The above-mentioned tests are the most commonly used by LLMDs. There have been others, such as a Lyme culture test developed by Dr. Joseph J. Burrascano. This test definitively indicated whether Lyme was found; however, it was limited in practice because it took more than a month for the culture to grow. At the time of writing, innovative tests are under development, such as metagenomic sequencing to identify Lyme bacteria and coinfections, and using bacteriophages, such as a test from a lab called R.E.D. Bacteriophages show promise as a way to determine the presence of different types of bacteria. The idea is to look for the bacteriophage instead of the bacteria itself. Bacteriophages are present only on active bacterial infections, so a phage-based test can be used as a proxy for an active infection (Shan et al. 2021).

ADDITIONAL SUPPORTING LABS

The following tests are often used to get a more general panorama for the individual's immune and toxic burden and are helpful for guiding treatment priorities. Although useful, many of the more functional tests are typically not covered by insurance.

Periodic Blood Work	Complete blood count (CBC). A skilled practitioner will be able to look at a standard blood panel and draw insights specific to Lyme and coinfections. (For example, seeing high or low neutrophil levels can be indicative of an active bacterial infection and a low RDW may be indicative of microbial activity.)
	A complete metabolic panel (CMP) is recommended throughout any treatment protocol to check liver and kidney function (as herbs and pharmaceutical interventions can affect their function).
Bioenergetic Testing	If no antibodies show up for Lyme coinfections, it doesn't mean you don't have them; it just could mean that the microbe is not primarily in the blood. According to biophoton physics, our cells communicate to each other through light, at the speed of light. Through this principle, bioenergetic testing can pick up on the presence of microbes, which communicate at a certain frequency, even when other labs and diagnostics fail. Although many of the following companies mention that this technique is not diagnostic per se, these tests analyze the energy that emanates from samples of hair, nails, saliva, or urine and can determine stressed or weakened digital values which serves as a proxy for various pathogens. Examples of energetic testing methods are the at-home kits from a company called Balanced Health, Electro-Acupuncture by Voll (EAV), and muscle testing, which is also described at length in the following section.
GI Health	The GI Map by Diagnostic Solutions indicates intestinal permeability otherwise known as "leaky gut" with a marker called zonulin, parasites, dysbiosis, secretory IgA, gluten sensitivity, and detoxification problems, like glucuronidation.
Inflammation Markers	CD57. These are called the natural killer type of white blood cells. They make up your innate immune system and fight infections like Lyme and even help to eliminate pre-cancerous cells. A low count can indicate chronic Lyme, and research has linked this marker to the probability of relapse (Stricker et al. 2002).
	C4A. A marker of inflammation and high also with mold illness.
Heavy Metals	A urine test to determine levels of excretion of heavy metals offered by Great Plains Laboratories.

Mold and Mycotoxins	RealTime Labs: urine test
	Great Plains Laboratories: urine test
	Mycotoxins: blood test for mycotoxins antibodies
Autoimmune Markers	There are many biomarkers that can indicate autoimmune tendencies, such as ANA, CRP, ESP, and thyroid antibodies along with a full thyroid panel including T3 and T4.
Organic Acids Test	Indicates how well metabolic pathways are performing. For the layperson, this test is hard to read, so you'll have to work with an experienced practitioner who is trained to interpret the results specifically for this test.
Genetic Testing	Although most people do not obtain actionable information to impact their protocols, some people find useful insights when working with a specialist. Genetic data from 23andMe can be analyzed with third-party services.
Nutrient Deficiencies	Both NutrEval and SpectraCell are blood tests to show nutrient deficiencies in detail.

PROVOCATION TESTING

Since Lyme and coinfections are not usually in the blood, many practitioners recommend a form of provocation; provoking the microbes to move and thereby become more accessible by testing methods. For example, provocation testing with urine samples involves lymph massage and ultrasound in order to drive out the spirochetes hiding in more stagnant tissues. Other approaches use systemic enzymes which can stimulate the release of spirochetes in the bloodstream with the idea of improving indirect testing by increasing IgM and IgG and also direct testing or PCR.

Another brute-force and simple way of determining problematic infections is through challenge testing where one uses remedies specific for each infection in hopes of provoking a reaction. Also, if you are unsure whether an infection is active or causing you symptoms, you can begin to treat it with the intention of provoking "die-off" or an increase in symptoms. These are herbal remedies that have minimal potential toxic effects in low dosage. However, the reader is encouraged to work with an experienced practitioner to determine a treatment plan.

ENERGETIC AND MUSCLE TESTING

In conventional orthopedics and neurology, muscle testing has been an important part of every physical exam to assess the health of the muscle itself or the nerve supplying it, often leading to further exploration via imaging techniques. However, when applied to complex chronic illnesses, it is powerful and sometimes indispensable when working through treatment to test the health of the autonomic nervous system, especially when combined with lab testing. Additionally, given the lack of accuracy of Lyme testing, muscle testing has earned its place in clinical practice when treating Lyme Disease.

Through muscle testing, you can determine which organs and organ systems are stressed, what infections you have using vials of the pathogens, and what supplements and medications are effective for you. You can throw a significant amount of money on doing functional lab testing; however, sometimes to guide treatment it can seem more like chasing a moving target. Muscle testing, on the other hand, allows you to get real-time feedback and have your body tell you which substances are helpful for you and which ones are not or could even be harmful. It seems almost too good to be true, yet it takes several years and much practice to be proficient at muscle testing. Good practitioners have decades of clinical experience behind them and are hard to find. Muscle testing can be extremely useful and even indispensable when guiding treatment as it extends beyond the limits of standard medical information gathering and gives immediate feedback anytime and anywhere you need it. Some people have gone to the length of learning forms of energetic testing to apply to their own healing as more and more courses are available online.

EAV is a bioenergetic testing modality and is an excellent alternative to muscle testing. Although not without its faults, EAV tends to be more objective in that it does not rely on the talent or experience of the practitioner. It is also called electrodermal testing (EDT), since when you are acutely stressed, sweat glands are activated and your skin becomes moist. There are newer systems using EDT from companies such as Avatar and Zyto. Although EDT minimizes the error of the practitioner, it is still not perfect and is subject to a margin of error with the amount of pressure applied and the sweat of the patient.

Since treatment is not a one size fits all, muscle testing can target a treatment plan to the individual person and their microbes. Multiple remedies may be recommended for coinfections, but different strains of these microbes may respond to only a subset of these remedies. Also, a person may respond better to another subset of remedies, so muscle testing helps make a protocol more effective and targeted. Also, the potency of herbs can vary across providers, so muscle testing can consolidate and verify dosing guidelines.

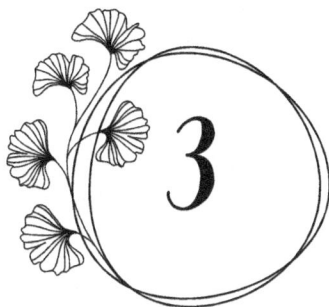

3

TREATMENT

As you can see from the previous two chapters, Lyme Disease is a politically and scientifically complex topic. Unfortunately, treatment is challenging and there is no one-size-fits-all solution. Practitioners are also varied in proficiency and can range from proponents of long-term pharmaceutical antibiotics to more holistic approaches. Many different protocols exist, such as Cowden, Klinghardt, Zang, and Buhner, and different combinations of antibiotics have different effects on the forms of the *Borrelia* bacteria, with some antibiotics forcing the bacteria to go into a persistent, harder-to-treat form (Cabello et al. 2017). For this reason, ILADS treatment guidelines include combination therapy with multiple types of antibiotics for chronic Lyme Disease (ILADS Working Group 2014).

Even before diving into killing Lyme and coinfections, you might need to address other bigger issues that impair immune function listed in the following chapter, such as parasites, mold, or candida. Conventional medicine looks for "one pill for an ill." However, chronic Lyme Disease involves many layers and many solutions that can be applied. Dr. Richard Horowitz, a pioneer in the field of clinical diagnosis and treatment of chronic Lyme, has developed a framework called multiple systemic infectious syndrome (MSIDS) for treating the patient more holistically and addressing what might be impairing the immune system so that it is better able to handle the Lyme.

WHY IS CHRONIC LYME HARD TO TREAT?

Lyme is one of the most genetically complicated bacteria. It has 132 genes, whereas for comparison, its cousin syphilis has only twenty. The Lyme bacteria can exist in multiple forms. Two of the bacterial forms are active and symptom producing. The first is the spirochete form, the spiral-shaped pathogen with an outer cell. The spirochete will grow and move throughout the body, and people experience this sensation as migrating symptoms, as the immune system responds to their activity. The second form is the cell-wall-deficient form which is sometimes referred to as the L form. The third form is called the cyst form which is dormant and not symptom producing. It has a dense outer wall that makes it resistant and impenetrable to antibiotics. More recently, a fourth form has emerged called biofilm. It is a structure created by different species of bacteria to control population growth, capture nutrients, and provide protection against assault. The spirochete colonies live in constant flux among these forms and each form requires a different antimicrobial medication for treatment.

An effective treatment protocol typically takes into account these multiple forms, and the morphing abilities of the Lyme bacteria addresses each coinfection individually. It is commonly thought that the biofilm makes Lyme difficult to treat as the bacteria may be susceptible to the antimicrobial but may be protected by a biofilm. Sometimes the process seems like a game of Whac-A-Mole, as coinfections can activate and reactivate. The most problematic and symptomatic infections can change, not to mention retroviruses and various other microbes and parasites may be transmitted as part of the same tick bite. It takes a skilled and experienced practitioner combined with an intuitive patient to navigate this dance and determine which infections are problematic and create an effective treatment plan. In fact, there is no one "cure," as Lyme Disease may be considered as a group of conditions: from retroviruses, infections from protozoa and bacteria, to even mold toxicity. If something works for you, it removes a layer that is causing you the most symptoms. Hence, the same protocol that gets someone else well might look totally different from the one that your body needs.

TREATMENT OPTIONS

"The journey of a thousand miles begins with one step."

—LAO TZU

Roughly half (52 percent) of the patients in the registry of MyLymeData undergoing treatment use antibiotics while others use a combination of alternative treatments (38 percent). So almost half the people report not taking antibiotics and 31 percent report using alternative treatments exclusively. For those who choose antibiotics, the treatment is typically targeted, long-course pharmaceutical antibiotics (Johnson 2019). This is not accepted practice by the CDC, Infectious Disease Society of America (IDSA), and insurance companies, but it's how many patients improve and is considered the standard treatment according to ILADS.

Furthermore, an unpublished study by the CDC states that the average duration is over 300 days and costs over $100,000 (Zhang et al. 2006). The toxicity and side effects of antibiotics are weighed against their benefit to kill the bacteria. You should work with doctors and specialists closely throughout the course of treatment to make sure that antibiotics are not causing additional harm. Some practitioners will treat the infection that causes most symptoms; others will treat in a specific order. Some practitioners pulse, which means antibiotics are applied for several days straight and then a break is given; others avoid pulsing with the reasoning that since *Bartonella* and *Babesia* replicate every twenty-four hours (whereas Lyme every four weeks or so). Also, these replication times are much slower than other bacterial infections, hence justifying longer-term treatment plans.

Fortunately, pharmaceutical antibiotics can be combined with herbal antibiotics and other alternative therapies. This book lists alternative or adjunctive treatment options in more detail, which can be added to a treatment protocol. Also, at the time of writing, a medication called Disulfiram—otherwise known as Antabus—has shown progress as an alternative to antibiotics, yet not without significant side effects and tradeoffs (Liegner 2019). Supportive oligonucleotide technique (SOT) is another emerging area that uses RNA segments to block the expression of segments of genes needed for Lyme or viruses to survive and replicate. Also, several antibiotics that have been recently identified and repurposed are undergoing trials to determine their efficacy for treating Lyme and coinfections.

HERBS OR PHARMACEUTICAL ANTIBIOTICS?

In a recent study published in *Frontiers in Medicine*, researchers from the Johns Hopkins Bloomberg School of Public Health analyzed the ability of fourteen plant-based extracts to kill *Borrelia burgdorferi*, compared to the currently used Lyme antibiotics doxycycline and cefuroxime. The researchers tested the effectiveness of these plant extracts in vitro and found that black walnut, cat's claw, sweet wormwood, Mediterranean rockrose, Chinese skullcap, and especially cryptolepis sanguinolenta and Japanese knotweed outperformed both antibiotics (Feng et al. 2020).

Lyme-practitioner approaches vary significantly on a spectrum of holistic to allopathic. However, in light of these findings, due to a less-toxic profile and efficacy demonstrated in studies many practitioners now opt to treat primarily with herbal protocols and incorporate pharmaceutical drugs only when warranted or only at the beginning of a protocol. Other practitioners have observed that treating Lyme with pharmaceutical antibiotics creates biofilms that allow microbes to go into a dormant state, not accessible by the immune system, which is not typically seen using herbs. Many practitioners have observed that this creates a situation harder to treat later; for this reason, they opt for herbal antibiotics instead.

The decision to use or not use pharmaceutical antibiotics is a personal one and depends on your circumstances. No one except you, with the help of your doctor, can judge what is the best option for your unique situation. The decision is also influenced by how symptomatic you are and how severely impacted your life is. If your symptoms are severe, then incorporating pharmaceutical antibiotics into your treatment protocol may be the best option, transitioning later to herbs.

If you are using herbs, make sure to work with an experienced practitioner who can help you understand interactions and synergies among different interventions and even better yet who can energetically test them for you. Just because these interventions are "natural" does not mean they do not deserve the same level of rigor when reviewing potential contraindications and interactions. For the intrepid reader, the book *Stockley's Herbal Medicines Interactions* is a good reference for checking these details (Williamson et al. 2019). Additionally, there are many books such as *Medical Herbalism* by David Hoffman if you're looking for a deeper dive into herbalism (2003).

PRECAUTIONS

One of the serious conditions that can occur with prolonged antibiotic use, and indeed an argument that's often used against long-term protocols, is called *Clostridium difficile* or *C. diff* where there is an overgrowth of bacteria that starts to produce toxins. Symptoms of *C. diff* are watery stools or diarrhea in addition to other GI symptoms, such as pain discomfort, bloating, cramps, and so forth. If you expect that you have *C. diff*, seek the help of a medical professional right away as it is a serious condition that needs to be treated promptly. The treatment is generally halting the current antibiotics and possibly starting a specific protocol to address the bacterial overgrowth. *C. diff* is not a frequent occurrence and you can decrease your chances by having a strong gut protocol on board, including taking a high-potency probiotic two hours before each antibiotic. Also, taking the probiotic strain *Saccharomyces boulardii* can help decrease your chances of developing and also ease a case of *C. diff*. The risk of *C. diff* is greater with pharmaceutical antibiotics than herbal antibiotics. So in cases where the infection is not acute (where there was not a definitive tick bite in a recent period of time), more and more practitioners opt for a herbal antibiotic approach due to the higher risk of these side effects.

Another serious consequence of prolonged antibiotic usage is overgrowth of yeast in the intestine. This condition is less immediately life threatening than *C. diff* but becomes problematic for recovery as it impairs immune function and is pervasive and hard to eliminate. There are also very limited tests for candida; however, if one takes multiple antibiotics for various months, it is a safe assumption that candida will develop even if the strongest probiotics are taken during treatment to protect the gut balance. Many candida symptoms mimic those of Lyme and can make your overall recovery slower. So wise practitioners will recommend a candida strategy, such as accompanying antibiotics with antifungals. Using antibiotics long term also damages mitochondria, which makes energy. Cells won't repair like they're supposed to and then the cell ceases to function when mitochondria don't function optimally. Sometimes it is also indicated to go off antibiotics and supplements with the guidance of your practitioner to give your body (and your liver) a break. Different combinations may have cumulative and synergistic effects when combined. More doesn't necessarily mean better.

Also, many people with Lyme end up being diagnosed with an autoimmune condition and prescribed immunosuppressants. However, immunosuppressants address the symptoms and not the root cause and suppress the immune system, which can potentially position patients for developing additional illnesses in the future.

HOW DO YOU KNOW THE TREATMENT IS WORKING?

Given the previously discussed problems with Lyme testing, unfortunately, there is no one-and-done test to definitively indicate if you are done with treatment. Most Lyme doctors will continue treatment once a patient is asymptomatic for several months. If a treatment is working, you should be able to see symptom improvement within two to three months. You might also use improvements in CD57 and C4A markers as indicators. Unlike other infections, with Lyme and coinfections, progression cannot necessarily be measured by seeing shifts in a decrease of IgM antibodies and an IgG increase (with the exception of *Babesia* specifically). As mentioned previously, there are also herbal tinctures that you can use to "test" for active infections. After sampling the tincture, if an increase of symptoms is induced, the infection is likely still problematic and is an indication of a need for further treatment. Muscle testing can also be helpful to determine if the infections are still creating stress on the body.

FLARE-UPS

Flare-ups or the dreaded herx reaction can happen during die-off when cytokines are produced in excess. This reaction or "healing crisis" can happen with microbial die-off caused by any kind of therapy from antibiotics to frequency-specific microcurrent (FSM). During these times, existing symptoms are increased and new symptoms can appear. To minimize the uncomfortable and sometimes debilitating experience, there are many recommendations that one can follow.

For example, during flare-ups, you can also alkalize your body as much as possible. There are many ways to alkalize the body ranging from breathing exercises, to drinking lemon water to baking soda or Alka-Seltzer Gold. Many people use Alka-Seltzer Gold, an over-the-counter medication typically used for relief for acid indigestion, heartburn, and sour stomach. However, it is advisable to take Alka-Seltzer Gold a few hours before or after taking antibiotics as it can affect their efficacy. Also, do not over-alkalize your body by taking more than several tablets of Alka-Seltzer Gold, as problems start to occur when your body becomes too alkaline. These should only be used sparingly and only when necessary. Also, don't take it within two hours before your next meal since it can affect the stomach acid which you need to help digest food. Using glutathione, the body's major antioxidant, along with its precursor NAC will help to ease the symptoms and help your liver detox. Liposomal glutathione, which is wrapped in fat for better absorption, may be helpful compared to other products that get broken down in the gut. Also, the herb Burbur made by Nutramedix drains your kidneys, liver, and lymphatic system quickly of toxins. When you get a herx reaction, put eight to ten drops in one-half cup of Burbur in water and drink every fifteen minutes. Within an hour or two, the herx will be greatly reduced. If you also want to detox your nervous system or when you are experiencing predominantly nervous system symptoms, then Burbur combined with another herb, Pinella, can be very effective.

Many people recognize herx reactions by a full-body pulsating sensation. Herx reactions can occur twenty-four to forty-eight hours after the antibiotic and can last weeks after. Sometimes they can also occur several weeks into treatment when an increased amount of die-off occurs. Sometimes herx reactions can be confused with detox reactions and medication side effects. Tune into your body, work closely with a knowledgeable practitioner, and learn how to distinguish from these two cases. You might need to pause your treatment to allow your body's detox capacity to catch up. Before doing so or making any changes in your treatment, consult your practitioner first. A good primary practitioner should have an emergency line available for escalated situations and should be able to guide you through escalated situations in treatment. Die-off reactions on the one hand mean that the treatment is working. However, on the other hand, they can be dangerous and have sent people to the emergency room.

During treatment, you may react to certain environments and experience allergy-like symptoms that you've never encountered before. You could be triggered by fluorescent lights, EMFs, or other environmental factors, such as chemicals and molds. This sensitivity will go away with successful treatment. However, in the meantime, you can just be aware that these sensations are happening and be in tune with your body. Also, with changes in elevation, many people experience an increase in symptoms. At higher elevations, with lower pressure and less oxygen, microbes are more active and able to replicate more readily. Given the option of living somewhere at sea level versus at a higher elevation, many, once they become aware of this difference, opt to live at a lower elevation at least for the duration of treatment. Hang in there and try to avoid environments that make you feel bad or uncomfortable and remind yourself that your heightened sensitivity will pass with treatment.

In the detox section of this book, many practices are listed to help during flare-ups, such as saunas, footbaths, castor-oil packs, and coffee enemas. Also, rest and recovery is paramount.

Be gentle with yourself. You also might need to put other life commitments on hold while you ride out more intense phases of treatment.

ROUTINE

During a flare-up or healing crisis, the importance of having a routine cannot be understated. Your routine or practice can be the compass in guiding you through hard times and maintaining balance. You can't change your external circumstances, whether a global pandemic or wildfire occurs for example, but you are 100 percent in control of your daily routine. Your fitness habits, the time when you eat and sleep, whether you have a morning routine or gratitude practice, all your activities and the priority you assign to them are entirely up to you. Also, sometimes you need to get out of your mind and into your body; a routine can help keep you on autopilot.

Although the following routine is specific for someone going through Lyme treatment and actively detoxing, after much repetition, it becomes automatic and can serve you for the rest of your life. Don't be hard on yourself if you don't check all the boxes all the time. Some days, when you are more symptomatic, just do what you're capable of. Here is an example of a routine that could be helpful while undergoing treatment:

- One glass of lemon water upon waking. Gargling with warm salt water to rebalance saliva pH.
- Oral health routine. If you have the practice, oil pull with either coconut or sesame oil for twenty minutes. If you're trying to remineralize your teeth, hold Quinton minerals in your mouth for a minute and then swallow.

- Sun gaze and get outside in the daylight or sunlight to reset circadian rhythm first thing in the morning.
- Get grounded with bare feet on grass and make contact with the earth. You can also use this opportunity to move your body, whether that means the five Tibetan rites, stretching, strength training, or yoga. Extra bonus points if you get dirty with mud on your skin for a healthy biome.
- If it's sunny outside, do this with the least amount of clothing possible for your body to synthesize the vitamin D from the sun. No matter how much vitamin D you take in via supplement form, you still need the sun for your body to activate it and make it available.
- Ice bath of 41°F–50°F for two to four minutes or a cold shower for activating your vagus nerve and decreasing systemic inflammation.
- Up until this time, you ideally haven't checked emails or used your phone to interact or receive messages as the nervous system is most raw in the morning.
- Rotate a detox methodology, either ionic footbath, sauna, coffee enema, castor-oil pack, and so forth.
- Take breaks from work throughout the day to keep up circulation and move lymph.
- Try to do something to support the liver every day, whether it is an herbal combination, a detox method, or even a simple castor-oil pack or liver-supporting food.
- Do some kind of exercise or movement, being mindful of what your body is asking for that day. If you have a wearable like an Oura ring, check it for guidance. Don't feel that you have to push yourself. Maybe you do 5 percent of what you used to do pre-Lyme and that's fine for now. Exercise has so many benefits from circulation to better sleep, so just

do something, whatever it is, and don't skip out on moving your body daily.

- Something to activate the parasympathetic nervous system. For example, meditation where you just focus on the breath. You can also incorporate prayer, gratitude, forgiveness, visualization, or whatever resonates or feels good for you in your current situation.
- Stop using digital products at 7:00 p.m., and start a winding-down routine, such as reading, writing, or yoga. This could include Epsom salt baths which help detox. Don't look at blue light, or if you need to look at screens, have blue-light-blocking glasses.

As you move through life, travel, and are around other people, things rub off on you and affect you in unexpected ways. Having a daily routine keeps you grounded and centered among all these forces that may affect you even without your knowing. Be intentional and plan your day around your well-being. Your habits and routine can arguably more directly affect your healing outcome than any pill or supplement you take.

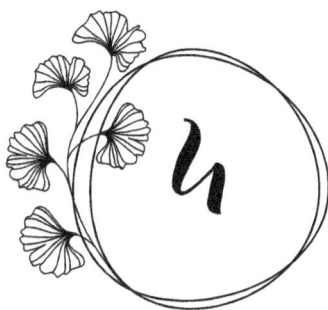

HEALING FACTORS

Stress, sleep, diet, environment, and mentality are pillars of your wellness and healing. Regardless of the treatment approach you choose, you already make hundreds of daily decisions on these factors which can have such a direct impact on healing. So what follows is a high-level summary of helpful tips and best practices on each topic as it relates to the specific challenges of Lyme.

STRESS

"Guard your heart above everything else, for from it flows all of the issues of life."

—KING SOLOMON, PROVERBS 4:23

Our ancestors from 200,000 years ago were not too biologically different from us in terms of our ability to manage stress. Thousands of years ago, the sympathetic nervous system, the fight-or-flight state, would have been activated only a small percentage of the time for our ancestors. A tiger appears. We run from the tiger and escape or die. The stressful event is over and we return to everyday life. Unfortunately, in today's modern world, we are "sympathetic dominant," meaning the reverse scenario is true where we might be in the sympathetic state 90 percent of the time. In an "always on" and connected world, sometimes we forget this. Compared to any other time in human history, humans have never before been under as much prolonged, chronic, and low-grade stress.

There are multiple studies in medical schools and institutions from Harvard to the Mayo Clinic that link stress to illness. Highly respected and renowned cellular biologist, Dr. Bruce Lipton at Stanford University, found that research indicates that over 95 percent of all illness occurs because of stress affecting the nervous system. According to Dr. Lipton, stress that produces physical symptoms is caused by deeply held beliefs about ourselves and our circumstances. These beliefs cause us to interpret our circumstances as a threat when in reality they are not. This misinterpretation is wired into us subconsciously and causes a chronic activation of the fight-or-flight response (Gustafson 2017).

Stress can impact our body in countless ways and affects our ability to heal. As long as you are constantly in stress, your body will respond according to the way it is programmed to do, deprioritizing digestive and reproductive function, adjusting cortisol levels, and diverting blood flow primarily to the muscles. Chronic stress decreases immune function, and over time, long-term stress can downregulate the healthy expression of genes. Stress also impairs natural killer cell function which is needed for fighting Lyme. It also increases a condition called mast cell activation where people can experience increased allergic reactions or overreactivity to certain environments or foods. In addition, stress decreases the integrity of the gut microbiome.

In summary, stress modulates the immune system so much that many people with Lyme have reported having flare-ups or even relapses when going through stressful life events. In fact, many Lyme patients are able to fight off the infection not realizing they have Lyme until a stressful event occurs in their life. Dealing with a chronic illness like Lyme where new symptoms come up constantly is stressful enough, not to mention the panic attacks or anxiety often accompanied by *Bartonella* and *Babesia* flare-ups. People who have never dealt with a panic attack may be taken off guard when the experience presents as a recurring symptom. Unfortunately, anxiety, if not dealt with, can be a roadblock to healing and keep a person in a disease state or mentality.

Stress can be measured objectively by heart rate variability, resting heart rate, and subjectively by tension and pain in different areas of the body. Also, on a brain map or EEG, you can measure brain wave activity to determine whether you are in a calm or anxious state of mind. If you have a Type A personality, the concept seems counterintuitive that relaxing is actually more productive to your healing. However, by being in a parasympathetic state more often, you are giving your body more opportunity to recover and detox. When we are in chronic stress, the sympathetic fight-or-flight state is activated. The parasympathetic on the other hand is achieved through sleep, meditation, savasana, and other activities that activate the parasympathetic nervous system.

So for this period in your life, you should be mindful of your sources of stress, either physical, mental, or emotional, and have a plan in place for managing stress and bringing your body into a parasympathetic state conducive to healing. For example, doing high-intensity interval training (HIIT) when your body is under physical stress or fasting when your adrenals are not functioning properly may not be the best choice. Listen to your body and be mindful while you are in treatment and healing. There are a number of herbal and botanical options that are helpful, such as passionflower, lemon balm, chamomile, magnesium, kava, CBD, and B vitamins, that can be very supportive of the adrenals and especially B6 for your nervous system.

Learn what works for you and have a strategy for entering into a parasympathetic state to calm the nervous system. If you are wondering where to start, here are a few specific practices and tools for stress reduction:

- **Emotional freedom technique (EFT).** This technique consists of tapping on acupressure meridians on the body to release blockages. The process starts with a beginning statement of what the problem, feeling, or emotion is and includes a complete acceptance and acknowledgment of the problem when the tapping is performed.
- **Nucalm.** This application uses proprietary software to generate binaural beats designed to move you from a stressed state (high beta range of 33–38 Hz) to the healing theta brain state, a more restorative state than sleep.
- **HeartMath.** This technique teaches you to alter your heart rhythm pattern primarily through deep breathing. Aware-

ness of breathing and heart rate then encourages a more relaxed state, which reduces stress and its side effects.

- **BrainTap.** A set of guided meditations meant to help you relax and activate alpha/theta brainwave states. The service comes with a headset that synchronizes light and sound and creates an immersed effect.
- **Apollo Neuro.** A wearable that uses vibration to calm your nervous system.
- **Relaxation response meditation.** An exercise that breaks the train of everyday thinking developed by Herbert Benson, MD. The exercise consists of repeating the same word or prayer on exhale for ten to fifteen minutes. If thoughts come up, simply say, "Oh well" and get back to the exercise. To get the full benefit, the exercise is recommended daily.

The above list is meant to provide inspiration if you don't already have a practice. Many of these tools incorporate a form of meditation, which is explained in the following section.

MEDITATION

The benefits of meditation are many and the evidence is strong and growing. It has been demonstrated study after study that meditation reduces stress and enhances overall well-being. Meditation helps calm your nervous system and allows your body to get into a restful and relaxation state so that it can repair itself. The rest that your body experiences in deep meditation is comparable to when you are asleep, as explained by Harvard cardiologist Herb Benson and Miriam Z. Keppler in *Relaxation Response* (1976).

Immunoglobulin A has been found to increase with meditation, which helps you defend against infection and viruses. Meditation also increases telomerase, an enzyme that helps rebuild the telomeres and releases gamma-aminobutyric acid (GABA), a chemical related to feelings of tranquility and calm, as well as serotonin. Meditation also kickstarts neuroplasticity which is the ability of our brain to reshape itself (Stapleton et al. 2020).

Meditation transforms brain waves into an alpha state, which is a relaxed and peaceful level of consciousness. According to extensive studies done by neuroscientist Dr. Jon Kabat-Zinn at the University of Massachusetts medical school, when you meditate, energy moves from the right frontal cortex, which is more active under stress, to the left frontal cortex, which is associated with calmness and less anxiety (*Full Catastrophe Living* 2013). Meditation also reduces the amount of activity in the amygdala, which is associated with fear.

Some people have used a visualization form of meditation to visualize their body in a healthy state using this technique so that the "body follows the mind." For those of us who struggle with quantifying the impact and progress, technology can give us feedback and track brain waves to determine whether we are in a calm state. The Muse headset is an at-home portable EEG device that gives real-time neurofeedback on how you are meditating. There are other meditation applications, such as an insight timer that is widely used and has a significant base of content.

Ultimately, the best meditation technique is the one you will adapt to and do on a recurring basis. However, learning with the help of a teacher or supporting yourself with an experienced practitioner will go a long way, both in providing guidance and accountability.

MOVEMENT AND FITNESS

"Illness loves stagnation."

—UNKNOWN

If we have well-functioning circulation and healthy bowel movements daily, we move through infections and toxins much quicker. Movement is especially important as it relates to the lymphatic system, since if you don't move, neither does your lymph, the colorless, watery fluid that contains white blood cells that attack the Lyme bacteria in the blood. The lymphatic system does not have a pump like the circulatory system does and relies on muscle contractions to pump lymph, which sends your immune soldiers around the body. If you are not moving, the lymph becomes stagnant along with your body's natural defenses and accumulates waste. This should be the number one takeaway from this section and indeed one of your main motivations to keep moving. Movement may not compare to a sexy therapy or supplement, but its impact is profound. In terms of its impact on the immune system, moderate exercise one hour a day for five days per week improves immune function. However, on the flipside, intense or strenuous exercise for two or more hours has been shown to actually decrease immune function.

Sometimes when we are tired and in pain, all we want to do is stay in bed. However, exercise will help to lower inflammation, facilitate detox, promote sleep, and also bring on a ton of other positive healing effects, such as increased endorphins. It helps drive Lyme bacteria out of the tissues where it is more readily available by the immune system. It cleanses the lymphatic system which removes waste, oxygenates tissue, helps the kidneys and gut. It is imperative that you get your lymph moving daily. A good reference point is walking for fifteen to twenty minutes minimum. Lyme Disease can affect the collagen fibers which can alter the healing of connective tissue—muscles, fascia, and ligaments. So exercise, even gentle movement, lubricates and hydrates tissues bringing in more nutrients for removing toxins.

An important part about exercising is not overexerting yourself as it will take you longer to recover and sometimes set you back in treatment. However, not exercising is not an ideal option. Even the smallest movements, such as walking or stretching, will go a long way. You might feel bad after exercising or on the following day, but this is not uncommon and means that your body is at work. Contrary to what some Lyme specialists say, you can do cardio, but be mindful of stress levels and adrenals. Aerobic exercise requires extensive amounts of oxygen that starve the yeast cells and kill candida growth. It also encourages neuroplasticity or neurogenesis—that is, new cells turning into neurons.

Walking outside has become a treatment in Japan called *shen ten yoku* or forest bathing. Just being, without doing anything, in nature is scientifically proven to lower heart rate, boost our immunity, increase a sense of contentment, connection, and creativity, and increases our sense of awe as described by Julia Plevin in *The Healing Magic of Forest Bathing* (2019). Being outside in the forest or by the ocean, now called "green or blue space" activities, has added multiple health benefits by exposing you to microbes from nature which diversify your microbiome along with negative ions that decrease inflammation. When we are inactive due to multiple symptoms, such as fatigue, pain, and weakness, we can age prematurely and that leads to a reduction in fitness and flexibility and thus a lower quality of life. Many people find that their recovery goes hand in hand with their fitness and often accelerates their fitness and recovery.

For all the above-mentioned reasons, it is critical that you move daily and have some routine to keep moving and exercising, however minimal you think it might be.

SLEEP

"Sleep is the best meditation."

—DALAI LAMA

Insomnia and sleep disturbances are one of the most common symptoms people with Lyme experience. Lack of sleep causes us to be grumpier, aggravates pain, worsens fatigue, increases inflammation, and further suppresses our immune system. Lyme generates an overproduction of cytokines in the sleep centers of the brain which creates a vicious cycle as sleep is needed to decrease cytokines. Sleep is where we spend one-third of our life, and many books have been written on the topic, such as *Why We Sleep*, which summarizes decades of sleep research (Walker 2017).

A challenge with correcting sleep problems is that there could be many reasons why your body is struggling to have restful sleep. You might also go through different phases where the root cause of your sleep problems changes. Many factors influence sleep, including infections, toxins, stress, hormonal imbalances, circadian rhythm imbalance, poor sleep hygiene, and environmental conditions, such as mold or EMF.

Sleep disturbances could be due to hormone imbalances; for example, you can have sleep issues at different times of the menstrual cycle or your problems could be due more to inflammation. With burned-out adrenals, cortisol levels may rise early in the morning to consistently wake you up or be abnormally high causing you trouble to fall asleep. Another common problem is inflammation or calming mast cells, so some people may find success if they deal with inflammation before bed. You might find yourself waking up and needing to eat, which could indicate a blood sugar regulation issue. Or it could be the persistent anxiety brought on by *Bartonella* or the panic attacks from *Babesia* that disrupt sleep. Maybe it was the late-night dinner that had sneaky gluten or night-shades that caused more inflammation than your body could handle. People become familiar with the gut-brain connection, since disturbances to the gut microbiome can disrupt sleep. Or maybe it is a full moon, and the increased parasite activity keeps you up. Also, if you find yourself consistently waking up at a certain hour throughout the night, in Chinese medicine, different times correspond to different organ systems; this could mean that an organ is stressed and needs more support.

Maybe your sleep disturbances are due to a combination of factors. Whatever the cause, people with Lyme struggle with sleep, yet proper sleep is indispensable for recovery. You should be getting between seven and nine hours of sleep every night. This point cannot be emphasized enough. People with Lyme must do what they need to do to prioritize sleep and must not sacrifice sleep for anything. Also, if taking an antimicrobial or supplement affects sleep, back off until you stabilize and regain reasonable sleep.

Sleep supports the immune system and gives you better pain control and more energy. If you are not getting enough sleep, prescription or herbal medicine should be used. The importance of good sleep for Lyme recovery, short and medium term, is likely outweighed by downsides or side effects of sleep medication.

There are many good resources out there for sleep hygiene; however, here is a summary of best practices and tips as it specifically relates to the challenges of Lyme:

- Avoid blue light from tablets, phones, or other screens in the evening as this light can be stimulating.
- If you have to stare at a screen with blue light three or four hours before sleeping, use blue-light-blocking glasses and a program called flux for your computer, which changes the screen lighting based on the time of day.
- Avoid caffeine, which has a long half-life that can also keep us up, and alcohol, which decreases deep sleep as our bodies may struggle to metabolize it.
- Minimize or eliminate cell phone and internet usage before bed as it is mentally stimulating.
- Keep your bedroom dark or use eye shades.
- Unplug your wireless router to reduce EMF exposure. A more extreme additional step would be turning off the circuit breaker in your house.
- During the day, use cold showers or plunges, working up

to two minutes each time, which helps bring down inflammation.

- Reset circadian rhythms by going outside first thing after waking up in the morning, which signals to your body that it is morning. Go outside without glasses and don't look through glass so that the blue light will not be filtered out and then look toward the sun. Even if the weather is cloudy or rainy, direct exposure to the morning light hitting your eyes sends a signal to your body and helps regulate circadian rhythm. Exposing yourself to light upon waking releases a healthy level of cortisol which acts as a wake-up signal, and it also starts an internal timer for the release of melatonin in the evening.
- Box breathing or extended box breathing can be helpful to enter into a parasympathetic state.
- Meditation apps, such as Insight Timer, Calm, or Headspace have guided meditation specifically for sleep that can be useful.
- Sometimes symptoms such as discomfort or pain from die-off can keep you up. In this case, alkalizing your body (using Alka-Seltzer Gold or baking soda) or binders can be helpful.
- Be asleep by 10:30 p.m. every night. Traditional Chinese medicine states that every hour of sleep before midnight is worth two hours of sleep after midnight.
- If you sleep with your partner, the reality might be that your sleep is optimal when you are both in separate beds, and at least for a period of time while you are recovering, you might need to sleep alone. This conversation might be difficult at first to have, but if you are well rested, you'll set the stage for better relationship health.

These are basic steps that anyone can take. However, additional measures can be made, such as converting your bedroom into a sleep sanctuary and EMF- and mold-protective space, as described in the related sections. Also, a great tracker for sleep and recovery is the Oura ring, which helps you track sleep quality as well as your overall readiness or ability to recover (it is recommended to keep any wearables in airplane mode to minimize EMF exposure). Sleep quality depends on a state called deep sleep, which is the restorative part and also helps with immune function, and the REM state which complements deep sleep.

Common supplements that can help are also listed below which ideally are taken an hour before going to sleep.

- **Curcumin or Quercetin.** Although not technically a sleep aid, these supplements help reduce inflammatory cytokines—small proteins released by the immune system as a result of the battle with the infections—and also calm mast cell issues. Cytokines are known to lessen the production of sleep-generating hormones in the brain. By taking curcumin throughout the day, you decrease inflammatory cytokines and lower inflammation in your body, setting up your body for the evening.
- **Phosphatidyl-serine.** A phospholipid or a fatty substance that acts as a protector of brain cells and a messenger among the cells. If you have high cortisol at night, this supplement may be helpful. Phosphatidyl-serine works to decrease the excess production of a particular hormone in the pituitary gland called ACTH, resulting in an overall reduction of cortisol levels in your body. When used at night, this supplement helps diminish stress and induce relaxation. Dosing recommendations depend on your bed-

time cortisol levels; however, typically a good guide is from 100 mg to 300 mg per night.

- **L-theanine.** This supplement is an amino acid that comes from green tea and assists in the formation of GABA, a calming, inhibitory neurotransmitter, which many people with Lyme are deficient in. L-theanine crosses the blood-brain barrier, which means it has a direct effect on your central nervous system; GABA is a necessary neurotransmitter for sleep. It is recommended to limit L-theanine to 800 mg per day.

- **5-HTP.** Your body uses this supplement to bolster the production of serotonin in the brain; a neurotransmitter that encourages relaxation and improves the quality of your sleep. As a word of caution, don't use 5-HTP if you are using other serotonin-boosting treatments, like certain antidepressants, anti-anxiety medications, and pain medications. Even though 5-HTP is natural, too much of a good thing—an overproduction of serotonin—can keep you wide awake.

- **Melatonin.** Some doctors recommend an initial dose of 0.5 mg—an amount that more closely mimics your body's natural production. However, some people seem to have trouble absorbing the supplement and benefit from higher doses, like the 1-, 3-, or even 5-milligram range. Melatonin also has an additional benefit that it detoxes the brain if used in liposomal form. Not a well-known fact, melatonin modulates our immune system, so sensitive people can actually feel an increase in symptoms when taking it. A helpful and better alternative for these people is using the slow-release type.

- **Magnesium glycinate.** Most people with Lyme are deficient in magnesium, which powers hundreds of reactions in our body. Although there are many forms of magnesium,

magnesium glycinate is one of the most absorbable forms. It promotes relaxation of your muscles and nervous system and helps you wind down before bed.

- **CBD or CBN.** Too much of the psychoactive component THC can be contraindicated in some people with an already overstimulated mind, and different strains can actually keep you awake. However, a small percentage of THC for the sedating effects is helpful as it promotes the "entourage effect," which means that the cannabinoid components are synergistic when combined together. CBN is also a sedating cannabinoid. Due to the lack of maturity of the cannabis industry, sourcing good-quality products is important as many products can be full of toxins and dirty terpenes.
- **Binders.** Although not meant as a sleep aid, nonstimulating binders can help mop up debris while going through detox or herx and can help ease symptoms when everything else fails.

Homeopathic remedies can also be helpful. There are a number of herbal and botanical options, such as valerian (practitioners observe that around 1 in 10 people can have an opposite effect of stimulation and agitation), passionflower, lemon balm, hops, and chamomile. The trouble with overuse of supplements, herbs, or pharmaceuticals and their combinations is overly suppressing the central nervous system. So use these supplements wisely and work with a practitioner who can guide you on their use. Although necessary in the short term to resolve insomnia and to help with recovery, in the long term, sleep aids should be reevaluated due to their negative side effects and also the ability to decrease the amount of REM and deep sleep. For example, with benzodiazepines, a type of prescription sleep medication, one should follow professional guidance with regard to their use, being weaned off the medication with a plan to gradually titrate down instead of stopping cold turkey which could cause rebound insomnia.

As you remove pathogens that can disrupt sleep, such as candida, parasites, Lyme, and fungi, sleep will come easier and improve. If the gut is weak, different nutrients and neurotransmitters are not produced. After exhausting many options and you still can't sleep, your body can recuperate to some degree if you rest and are still, as if you were asleep such as in a guided meditation or yoga nidra session, which can help your body rest when you can't sleep. Finally, lack of sleep can also be your body's way of telling you that you need to change course or perhaps back off on killing microbes or even make lifestyle changes.

For those who struggle with the spiritual questions around sleep and are curious to explore its deeper purpose, readers are encouraged to check out *Hush: A Book of Bedtime Contemplation* by Rubin Naiman, PhD (2014).

NUTRITION

"Let food be thy medicine, and let medicine be thy food."
—HIPPOCRATES

This quote stands the test of time. In herbal medicine, there is little distinction between food and medicine. During a healing journey, your body needs you to show up to your plate in the right way, because diet will significantly impact your healing journey and recovery. What you put in your mouth either helps or hurts you. Your diet can help you just as much as any supplement regimen can, so try to think of your diet as just that—a way to meet nutrient deficiencies and help your body get through this current phase of healing. Choosing what you put into your mouth can be extremely confusing and stressful, especially when it causes you to feel worse. Although the information that follows is dense, I've done my best to highlight the main points without going down too many rabbit holes.

Based on nutritional imbalances, you may need to change your diet. Lyme, parasites, and other pathogens can steal nutrients from you. You can use blood tests, such as NutrEval and SpectraCell, or energetic scans, such as the OligoScan, to determine deficiencies. People with Lyme are typically deficient in B6 and magnesium. You may find that through diet alone, you are not able to address deficiencies and need to supplement. With supplements, go low and slow; work up to the dose as your body may react to some minerals or binders. Some people find that a B vitamin can be helpful in the case of detoxing challenges or with a genetic MTHFR mutation. Consider that your nervous system also needs protein (typically 20 g of protein per meal), omega-3 fats, and magnesium. The book *Lyme Diet* goes into more detail on the specifics to nourish and repair specifically for people with Lyme (McFadzean 2010).

A low-inflammatory and alkaline diet using generally a paleo-type approach works well for many people. An autoimmune diet is optimal but more restrictive. To get some quick wins, eliminate sugar, dairy, and gluten. There are many reasons to avoid sugar. Sugar decreases your white blood cell count by 80 percent within four to five hours after eating it (Ullah Janjua et al. 2016). Lyme bacteria also feed on sugar, so eliminating concentrated sources of it is a basic first step. For you, this change may or may not mean reducing natural sugar sources and fruit. Many people with Lyme avoid a carb-heavy diet and have seen success incorporating healthy fats following a more keto-type diet. A strict keto diet over time can put too much stress on the liver, gallbladder, and adrenals. However, a rotating keto diet is recommended, such as the version refined by Dr. Terry Wahls and Eve Adamson (*The Wahls Protocol* 2014). Before going keto, it is recommended to do a full thyroid blood panel and also gauge digestion, as sometimes following a ketogenic diet without enough stomach acid could cause digestion problems, and not eating enough carbs can also interfere with sleep. Also, an alkaline diet will help you through flare-ups and can ease symptoms (Young and Young 2002). Between meals, you may drink lemon water, since lemons have an alkaline effect once in your body. To determine your alkalinity, you can use pH strips which change color based on the alkalinity of your urine. Another consideration is a lectin-avoidance diet. Grains, nuts, beans, and seeds all contain lectins, which are essentially a poison from the reproductive part of a plant. Foods with phytic acid, for instance grains, beans, seeds, and nuts, should be organically grown and then soaked in water or fermented before eating. Phytic acid blocks mineral absorption as it tightly binds phosphorus and blocks its bioavailability. It can also bind and block zinc, calcium, and iron. Pressure cooking and soaking these foods for at least twenty-four hours starts a germination process and addresses the issue. If these measures are not followed, a lectin-avoidance diet is a consideration. Also, companies such as Eden Organics sell beans and seed products prepared this way already. It is also recommended to minimize or take extra caution with seafood for potential metal exposure. The bigger the fish, such as tuna and swordfish, the more potential for contaminants. On the other hand, wild salmon and sardines can be safe options. Try to eat or drink as much fresh herbs as you can. One commonality in the blue zones, areas studied around the world with the highest concentration of centenarians, is the abundant consumption of herbs. So make cilantro or parsley dips, or throw rosemary into your juicer. There are also many herbs and spices that you can incorporate to help boost immune function. For example, medicinal mushrooms such as reishi, turkey tail, and cordyceps can support your immune system, especially for their ability to increase globulin, affecting immunoglobulin and ultimately WBC count. Another consideration in reducing the overall body burden through diet is oxalates, which are a protective mechanism of a plant and are responsible for causing crystallization in different parts in the body, with the most infamous manifestation being kidney stones. Some people may be more genetically susceptible than others. Oxalates are quite ubiquitous, so rather than avoiding them completely, one can pay attention to the foods with the highest concentration. Typically, the biggest offenders are:

- Spinach
- Swiss chard
- Most nuts like cashews, almonds, and Brazil nuts
- Rhubarb
- Cacao

Including sources of calcium in a meal can aid with binding and removing the oxalates, thereby reducing their damaging effect, while some people proactively take herbs like stone breaker.

These dietary considerations from oxalates, lectins, to keto and paleo may seem overwhelming, so try different changes and check in with how your body feels. In terms of more general considerations, here is a summary of the top recommendations:

- Avoid your food sensitivities. There are numerous lab tests to look for food allergies and intolerances (IgE, IgA, IgG, cytokine reactions, Type IV allergies, and more). Muscle testing or energetic testing can be helpful. Muscle testing can indicate food intolerances but will indicate which foods act as medicine and are healing. For most people, this means avoiding dairy, gluten, and sugar. Also, while your gut is still repairing, it is advised to avoid nightshade vegetables like peppers, potatoes, tomatoes, and eggplant.
- Avoid eating burned or smoked food.
- Wash vegetables in baking soda or apple cider vinegar to clean for any parasites.
- Avoid all vegetable oils and their polyunsaturated fatty acids including soybean, corn, and canola, which are inflammatory.
- Before eating, activate the parasympathetic nervous system so you are in a more relaxed state and more nutrients are readily absorbed from the food. Whatever works for you, be grateful, pray, or meditate briefly.
- Make sure your cookware and utensils are not toxic. Many nonstick cookware products are mostly toxic, and safer options exist such as those from companies like Extrema.oh
- Avoid monotony. Rotation and breadth are good guiding principles to go by. Eat a variety of foods to nourish your gut microbiome and frequently rotate. A great benchmark would be to try to eat at least thirty types of vegetables per week.
- Be mindful that leftover food is more likely to develop mold.

- Optimize for eating as many plants as possible for their associated phytochemicals.
- All grains and beans must be soaked to remove phytic acid.
- Incorporate mineral-rich herbs in pesto or teas.
- Eat vegetables that are organic and grown in mineral-rich soils. Inorganic food has more glyphosate, in particular soy, wheat, and corn. If eating organic is not possible and the quality of food is questionable, there are different remedies you can take to neutralize any possible glyphosate, such as peat extract.
- Eat local and seasonal so that the nutrient content is higher. Vegetables when harvested before they are ready lose significant nutrient content.
- Chewing food slowly allows saliva to be released in the mouth and mix more thoroughly with the food and with amylase, the enzyme in saliva to help with digestion.
- Be mindful of food combinations. For example, don't eat fruit with a big meal.
- Do not drink right after eating.

The last few points are from ayurveda, which people can find useful for balancing diet to the needs of the body and also adapting to seasonal and environmental changes. In ayurveda, "you are what you digest," not what you eat. Standing on the shoulders of traditional wisdom and practices like ayurveda can serve as a very relevant and time-tested guide to balanced healthy living. For a good summary, refer to *Living Ayurveda: Nourishing Body and Mind through Seasonal Recipes, Rituals, and Yoga* (Ragozzino 2020).

One of the most common mistakes people can make is to become too restrictive. Over time, this tendency toward *orth-*

orexia, or an obsession with restricting certain foods, creates deficiencies or imbalances in certain nutrients. Keep in mind that dietary changes are temporary to get you through a certain phase or to lower inflammation. They are a tool in the toolbox but don't have to be a lifelong constraint. Eating for joy and pleasure is also part of being healthy and too much restriction for too long can become a source of stress. As you feel better and recover, you can try slowly introducing other foods, for example incorporating noninflammatory grass-fed dairy. Neuroplasticity described in the following chapters may also play a part in whether you react to certain foods.

As you get better, you can rely less on supplements and more on whole food sources for your nutrition. For example, for copper, try oysters, liver, spirulina, or other algae. Whole food sources also provide you with the full spectrum of compounds. For example, instead of ascorbic acid (which over time can cause imbalances), consume foods high in vitamin C like berries, citrus fruits, and broccoli which provide bioflavonoids and antioxidants as well as all the other vitamin C constituents.

As we've reviewed, what you put in your mouth, how it is prepared, and where it comes from can have profound impacts on your healing. The information presented here might be overwhelming and even contradictory. Do not stress. Your nutritional needs will also change throughout your journey. So start wherever you are and know that this knowledge will serve you for the rest of your life, and many practices you will continue to use even after you recover.

WATER

The water you drink becomes your blood. Let that sink in for a moment. Improving your water is one of the most powerful and direct upgrades you can make for your health. Water is the basis of all life and that includes your body. Your muscles that move your body are 75 percent water; your blood that transports nutrients is 82 percent water; your lungs are 90 percent water; your brain that is the control center of your body is 76 percent water; even your bones are 25 percent water.

So maybe one of the best investments you can make in your health is being selective about your water. Unfortunately, much municipal water has fluoride, chlorine, and many inorganic and organic substances that aren't filtered out, such as used pharmaceuticals. Carbon filters are insufficient as a stand-alone filter and produce acidic water with contaminants. Spring water is excellent as natural aquifers add fulvic acid and minerals which the body uses. Spring water contains amounts of natural silica which helps eliminate unwanted aluminum from your body. You can find a spring near you in the United States using the site findaspring.com. If you don't have access to spring water, a high-quality filter like Berkey is a good option. However, tap water filtered through Berkey is still considered hard water as it contains a high enough "total dissolved solids" or TDS reading. When comparing all these alternatives, if you do not have access to spring water reverse osmosis or distilled water is best. Reverse-osmosis systems can be purchased to integrate with your kitchen or simply as a countertop filter. Although reverse osmosis is ultimately the best option, it lacks minerals. So adding electrolytes and deep sea minerals such as Quinton is advisable as the adrenals, which are often low functioning in people with Lyme, regulate the balance between sodium and potassium. Brands like Fiji in the United States and Acilis in Europe have amounts of silica, an important trace mineral for strength and flexibility of the connective tissues of your body like cartilage, tendons, skin, bone, teeth, hair, and blood vessels.

ENVIRONMENT
EVERYDAY TOXINS

Many practitioners use the analogy of a bucket to describe someone's overall load of toxins. As you empty the bucket or toxic body burden through detox and address pathogens, you also want to decrease the amount of toxins going into the bucket. Unfortunately in today's environment compared to fifty years ago, this task is becoming more challenging.

In the late 1940s, the chemical age took off, fueled by technology developed during World War II. Before this time, virtually no petroleum-based pesticides and few petroleum-based household products had been in use. Now today, more than 5 million chemicals are known worldwide, and unfortunately, we know very little about the toxic effects of the great majority of these chemicals (Schafer et al. 2004). A National Research Council study found that complete information on the hazards to human health was available for only 10 percent of pesticides and for only 18 percent of chemically derived medication (Dadd 1990, 7).

In 2010, approximately 80,000 chemicals were found on the market in the United States, many of which are used by millions of Americans daily, and they're un- or understudied and largely unregulated (Reuben 2010). According to worldometers. info, approximately 10,000,000 tons of chemicals are released into our environment each year. Of these, over 2,000,000 tons per year are recognized as carcinogens ("Environment" 2022). On top of these environmental factors, in today's age, our buckets are already quite full when we come into the world. A 2005 study by the Environmental Working Group highlights how toxic the current environment is. Researchers from this study tested umbilical cord blood—that is, the blood that is pumped back and forth between the placenta and a developing fetus— for toxicity. It was found that the cord blood now contains at least 287 industrial chemicals. Of the chemicals detected, 180 are linked to cancer in humans or animals, 217 are toxic to the brain and nervous system, and 208 cause birth defects or abnormal development in animal tests (Houlihan et al. 2005).

Indeed, we have never before in history had to face such an enormous toxic hurdle starting from infancy. Over a lifetime, many factors accumulate and add to one's toxic load: heavy metals and aluminum in the air, amalgam fillings, chemicals in our food and water, such as glyphosate, fluoride, and PBDEs, xenobiotics such as bisphenol A, and hormonal residues from drinking water, solvents, biotoxins from microorganisms, mold, parasites, and internal infections, metal implants, material breast augmentation or other surgeries, silicone, tattoos, home and workplace exposures such as leaded paint, dust, formaldehyde, and gasoline, and so forth. The list goes on. Among the biggest perpetrators, many practitioners identify a few factors including but not limited to iron overload, glyphosate, aluminum, and polyunsaturated fats as significant contributors to dysregulation in the body and chronic illness.

Making changes to reduce toxic exposure can be overwhelming. So where does one start? Replacing toxic cosmetics and soaps with petroleum-free alternatives is a simple step and can be done immediately. Replacing your kitchen cookware along with cleaning and personal products may seem like a costly, daunting task, but it is a small price to pay when considering the positive impact in lowering your toxicity burden over time. Small daily actions can have a huge impact. For example, avoid chemicals such as perfumes, insecticides, pesticides, fabric softeners, household cleaning products, and air fresheners. Do not use aluminum-based antiperspirants. If you smoke, you should quit as your body has enough to do without having to detox these chemicals as well. If you have to handle strong chemicals for some reason, use gloves and a mask. Also, it is a good idea to invest in shower filters, such as those from companies PH Prescription or Live Pristine, for example. Many toxins, such as fluoride and prescription medicine residues from municipal water supplies are absorbed through our skin.

EMF

In addition to the inorganic and organic chemicals, the body is exposed to energetic toxins. One topic that has gained popularity in recent years is the topic of electromagnetic frequencies (EMFs).

However, EMFs are not new and have always affected us, from the EMF from the sun to the electromagnetic pull from the earth. In fact, the reality is that we are bioelectric human beings. We have an electric frequency that we emit, and each of our organs has a specific frequency. It has been measured that the heart had a strong field that emits eight feet out from the body. However, when it comes to damaging electromagnetic waves, it's the higher frequency that can be more troublesome as shown below.

THE ELECTROMAGNETIC SPECTRUM

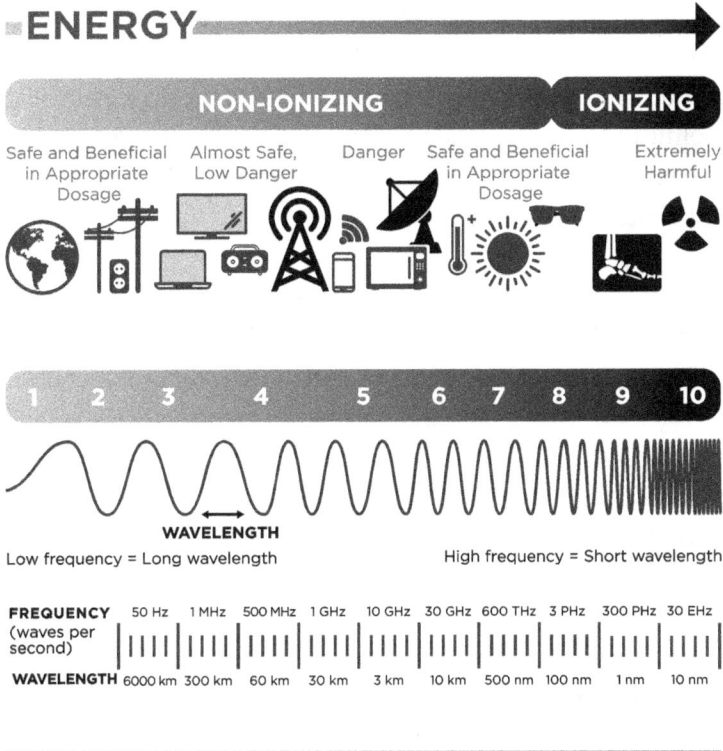

ENERGY ➡️

NON-IONIZING				IONIZING

Safe and Beneficial in Appropriate Dosage	Almost Safe, Low Danger	Danger	Safe and Beneficial in Appropriate Dosage	Extremely Harmful

1	2	3	4	5	6	7	8	9	10

WAVELENGTH

Low frequency = Long wavelength   High frequency = Short wavelength

FREQUENCY (waves per second)	50 Hz	1 MHz	500 MHz	1 GHz	10 GHz	30 GHz	600 THz	3 PHz	300 PHz	30 EHz
WAVELENGTH	6000 km	300 km	60 km	30 km	3 km	10 km	500 nm	100 nm	1 nm	10 nm

1. Extremely Low Frequency   **5.** Microwaves   **8.** Ultraviolet
2. Very Low Frequency   **6.** Infrared   **9.** X-Ray
3. Low Frequency   **7.** Visible   **10.** Gamma Rays
4. Radiofrequencies

However, when referring to EMF exposure, we often refer to non-native EMF—that is, man-made or not native to humans— such as those from high-tension wires, power transformers, fluorescent lighting, electric and hybrid vehicles, computers, and other electronics, such as cell phones and portable music players. When using the term *EMF* in this section, it is intended to refer to these non-native EMFs. Our exposure to these sources has increased exponentially in the last few decades. For example, the average American has thirteen different wireless devices in their home, from cell phones, tablets, to all sorts of connected appliances, which are all sources of electrical pollution. Our wireless connectedness has only emerged in recent years of human history, and we are only beginning to understand the implications.

It is often cited within the telecom industry that the radiation from Wi-Fi and phone signals are low energy and not ionizing. So it is not damaging our DNA directly and it cannot break molecular bonds and harm us in the way that X-rays or microwaves do. However, according to Dr. Martin Pall from Washington State University, the main mechanism of harm is actually how it impacts our "voltage-gated channels," which increases calcium in our cells. Too much calcium inside the cell is not good as it creates oxidative damage and decreases energy production by affecting the mitochondria (Pall 2018). When non-native EMFs open voltage-gated calcium channels, iron also goes into the cell together with calcium. Magnesium is a calcium blocker, so it is recommended to check magnesium levels if non-native EMFs are a concern.

As early as 1990 after hundreds of studies, the EPA recommended that these types of EMF be classified as a class-B carcinogen—that is, probable of causing cancer. However, after significant pressure from lobbyists, the EPA decided to take back this decision. Studies have shown that these EMFs are responsible for a twofold to threefold increase in cancer rates of children exposed to them particularly in terms of leukemia, lymphoma, and brain tumors (Pall 2018; Levitt 1995). Other studies have been shown to affect the size of the thymus gland and white blood cell count. In addition, in people who experience heightened mast cell activity, EMFs can aggravate the situation. For example, just being in the presence of a cell phone will activate the mast cells significantly and cause related symptoms.

With Lyme, EMFs are troublesome due to their impact on our microbes. Many practitioners believe that non-native EMF smog causes the microbes within us to believe they are under attack. This effect is a stressor for them, and they respond with the only mechanism they have by creating more biotoxins. For everyone, but especially for those with neurological symptoms, EMF remediation alone may have a significant impact on reducing symptoms.

Although we can't avoid high-energy, non-native EMFs completely, there are basic steps we can take to minimize their potential negative impact while we are still healing and feel more affected by them:

- Don't hold your phone up to your head. Use a speakerphone or headset. When using the speakerphone option, hold the phone at least six inches away from your head while making a call. Another option is to use a well-shielded headset with an air tube so that there is no wire going up to your head.
- Hardwire your internet and use Ethernet cables. Also, for the interested readers, you can hardwire your phone when you need to take calls and don't have your computer.
- Try not to put your phone in your pocket right up against your skin.

- When not using your phone, turn it on airplane mode (making sure that the four antennas, GPS, Wi-Fi, Bluetooth, and cellular data are all off).
- When you go to bed, turn it on airplane mode and don't have it charging right beside your bed. Phones that are charging emit up to ten times as much EMF.
- Don't use your laptop while it is charging.
- Turn off your Wi-Fi at night.
- If you are among the more sensitive, look into EMF-protective clothing (especially when flying) and faraday cages for bed canopies.
- Use a faraday cage around your router and make sure that the router is not in your bedroom or within ten feet of your bedroom. Connect the router to a plugin timer so that it turns off at night. Especially important is making sure you are protected when sleeping.

Ultimately, the measures you take are up to you. Remember that your cumulative EMF load is what matters, yet your body is resilient (DeBaun and DeBaun 2017). In addition to the steps mentioned above, many people go to additional measures to create a "sleep sanctuary," given how important sleep is for recovery as described in previous sections. Most people won't need or want to go to these measures; however, they are listed here for the interested reader.

- Use beds without metal as metal frames and metal box springs may amplify and distort earth's natural magnetic field.
- Use battery clocks near the bed as many electric clocks can produce high magnetic fields.
- Turn off bedroom circuit breakers.

- Use the filters on outlets called Stetzer filters.
- Make sure there are no elevated magnetic fields. Magnetic fields from appliances and building wiring can penetrate walls into a bedroom and disrupt the body's communication system. Special paints such as the product YShield provide an electro-conductive coating for the protection against a range of electric fields.
- On some phones you can deactivate 5G and 4G depending on what phone you use and where you are.
- Invest in a bed canopy. There are manufacturers such as slt.co.

Cleaning up electropollution can be overwhelming as EMFs are everywhere. For more resources, *The Non-Tinfoil Guide to EMFs* by Nicolas Pineault is an easy read and practical guide (Pineault 2019). Generally, the more densely populated the area or city, the higher exposure to non-native EMF. So depending on where you live, your exposure will be different. In terms of priorities, you should be cleaning up what is in your bedroom and then in your home. You can also more precisely measure EMF stress in your environment with a simple gauge. The EPA has set a safety level no greater than 1 mG (milligauss). However, many functional doctors, like Dr. Joseph Mercola, have recommended that ideally EMFs should not exceed 0.5 mG as a precaution (2008). Beyond your home environment, Antennasearch.com is a good resource to learn where cell towers are in your neighborhood.

Apart from these measures, there are also additional supplements that may be helpful along with creams and protective clothing. When you travel via plane or a long drive, it is recommended to use precautions with EMF-protective clothing lined with silver. As you decrease your heavy metal and microbial burden, you may find yourself less sensitive to EMF. Also, different genetics can increase susceptibility.

Among the toxins we live among, EMF affects humans and other microbes in ways we are still learning to quantify. Depending on who you ask, practitioners have varied opinions as to their impact on people with Lyme, with some practitioners refusing to treat people who are not EMF aware to others who do not factor it into a treatment plan. Whether this section resonates with you (pun intended), the good news is that there are many simple ways to protect yourself and be mindful of how certain non-native EMFs affect us.

PSYCHO-EMOTIONAL

"You cannot separate mind from body."

—SOCRATES

Our physical bodies can be a barometer for our inner health. Yet many people leave the emotional or mental part of healing last and later regret not prioritizing it earlier. Many savvy practitioners and people who have been through a healing process can attest to the impact of the mind-body connection and consider spiritual, emotional, mental, and energetic factors into the recovery process.

Everyone deals with the mental and emotional part of healing, and in some cases, it can set the stage for the illness. Even going through a complicated illness like Lyme can be a trauma in and of itself. Around 12,000 years ago, Patanjali, who wrote the yoga sutras and created the foundation for modern-day yoga, knew the importance of the mind-body connection and determined that we are much more than just the physical body. He believed that we are made up of multiple layers. We've recognized this complexity of the human experience thousands of years across cultures, and modern research has brought insights to light. An emerging field called psychoneuroimmunology is getting more attention and producing more studies. Indeed, emotions influence the immune system in ways we are only beginning to understand as described beautifully in *Molecules of Emotion* and *Biology of Belief* (Pert 1997; Lipton 2005). From the lens of psychoneuroimmunology, our body is a pharmacy capable of producing all sorts of biochemicals conducive to healing. Two areas that can have a significant impact for the healing process are community and mindset.

COMMUNITY

Dr. Vivek Murthy, surgeon general of the United States, famously said that loneliness is more deadly than smoking a pack of cigarettes. Many people with Lyme can feel lonely and isolated as the disease may not be well understood by close family members or friends. Sometimes when we feel sick, we just want to crawl up in a ball and be alone. However, it is a sense of isolation and loneliness that makes the journey even more challenging.

The positive impact of being surrounded by a support network has been quantified in many studies. For example, one case is the town of Roseto in Pennsylvania in the 1960s which had half the national average for heart disease. Researchers performed a study to determine the root causes for this anomaly. From 1900 to 1960, society there emphasized community and the church. As a result, the sense of safety was more palpable in daily life (Gutkin 2009). Researchers found that how we retrain our immune system to feel safe is extremely important for overall health. If a child had a problem in these supportive societies, they went to a neighbor or community leader for help. The sense of extended family is not the same as it was several decades ago. Today, most people in modern society don't have safety nets. Instead, we live in nuclear families and don't support ourselves from our extended community relationships. Since the study of Roseto in Pennsylvania, more research has surfaced.

A study by NASA found that when humans are socially isolated in a monotonous environment, the hippocampal part of the brain shrinks (2020). Feelings of loneliness cause physiological changes in the body. This book was written during the height of the coronavirus pandemic during public quarantines when more studies were done in the area (Choukér and Stahn 2020). According to the polyvagal theory, we are social beings, and we do need to be supported by other human beings to heal. As human beings, we crave connection. Multiple studies show the benefits of hugging and human connection, as hugging increases oxytocin levels in the body. In the same study, women also saw positive effects of oxytocin when they held their infants closely (Light et al. 2005).

Find a community that gives you energy or try to maintain a connection with one that you already have. Surround yourself with positive influences for your healing, people who bring you up and are empathic to your situation. You are not alone in this journey, and there are many wonderful human beings who can help.

MINDSET

Many aspects of your experience being sick up until now may seem unfair—from the diagnostic tools that are at best half-effective, to the disconnected, conventional medical community that treats Lyme as taboo, to the unclear and at times excruciating and ineffective treatments. On top of dealing with a traumatic process to find a diagnosis, by now you are used to the challenge and the complexities of navigating this illness. Chronic Lyme Disease can mean huge changes in quality of life; it can affect family dynamics and your ability to work. Healing is a marathon, not a sprint, and can put a strain on relationships over time.

You will also have a thousand reasons why the current situation of Lyme Disease is unfair. Indeed the state of tick-borne infection awareness, treatment, and therapeutics are way behind where they need to be, and conventional medicine has to catch up. However, adopting a victim mentality will not be helpful and may even get in the way of your recovery. Also, identifying with the illness and blaming others may provide some relief in the short term but will not ultimately be productive.

The effects of our mind on our physical experience are well documented with the concept of placebo. The power of placebo got steam in World War II when medical staff ran out of morphine, so doctors and nurses used a vial with saline solution. When they used it on patients saying that it was pain-killing morphine, doctors observed that patients experienced relief. Today, much work has been done, especially in the emerging field of psychoneuroimmunology, to explain the role of placebo since a landmark study published fifty years ago claimed that placebos can affect patient outcomes at least 35 percent of the time (Beecher 1955).

More recently, there was a series of experiments with elected surgeries in 2002 where a control group went through everything that the actual surgery group did including fasting, anesthesia, and receiving real surgical incisions, yet they didn't actually receive the procedure itself. Many patients in the control group, who were unaware that they did not receive the actual procedure itself, experienced a relief in symptoms and deemed the surgery a success. In fact, in about half of the cases, the fake surgeries worked as well as the actual surgeries (Moseley et al. 2002). These experiments were later canceled.

A later review in 2014 of placebo-controlled trials found that placebo led to improvements 74 percent of the time while 51 percent of the time, placebo effects did not differ to those from surgery (Wartolowska).

For example, a 2010 meta study looked at 202 drug trials where a placebo group was compared to patients who received neither placebo nor active drug and found that placebos can even improve outcomes for pain, nausea, asthma, and phobias (Hróbjartsson and Gøtzsche).

Placebos have also been found to decrease symptoms conditions such as Parkinson's disease, fatigue depression, and anxiety (Lieberman et al. 2004).

Additionally, doctors acknowledge the importance of placebo. Researchers at the National Institute of Health surveyed 679 internists and rheumatologists. Of those doctors, 62 percent believed that using a placebo treatment was ethically acceptable and more than half reported using placebos in their practice (Tilburt et al. 2008).

Multiple books have been written on the topic of spontaneous remission documenting thousands of individual cases of people who have been cured or are in remission thinking they took medication, while in reality they were in the control group. On the flipside of this perspective, the nocebo effect can be profound as it affects negative thinking. In other words, how one perceives a treatment or even the projection of a doctor's attitude can affect the outcome of a protocol.

Where your attention flows, energy goes. If you believe you are sick and focus obsessively on symptoms, that's what your body and mind will prioritize and send energy to. Conversely, if you put yourself in a state where you see yourself healthy and well, you will set yourself up to get there. So throughout your healing journey, instead of focusing on what is wrong—negativity biases the brain to focus on things that are going wrong—look at what is going right. When making decisions, think about what the "healthy" version of you would do and let that mentality guide you, to the extent that it is reasonable and practical to do so. Cultivate this mindset as you progress in your healing journey and you will benefit in many ways, including encouraging neuroplasticity and triggering your body's own healing mechanisms.

In summary, anyone who has been through a healing process will attest to the power of the mind in different ways and understands that the nonphysical can manifest in physical symptoms. Following this line of thinking, the word *patient* was later replaced throughout this book intentionally. Some people have found that only when ceasing to think of themselves as a patient and reframing their health around more positive states of well-being as opposed to attacking pathogens, infections, and illness did they move past a disease state and experience real healing. Others have found a shift in perspective of assuming responsibility helpful. When people are sick, they depend on other people, not unlike how children rely on elders. Some people remain chronically sick because they are able to escape reality this way and at some level, they are not ready to be healthy. The previous concept may be hard to accept, or on the other hand, it may not resonate with you at all.

5

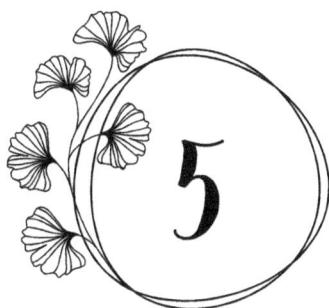

IMMUNE FUNCTION

Your body wants to be in good health and it wants to get back into balance. This chapter is about giving your body what it needs to support your immune system so it can better deal with Lyme. Often, the root cause of the person's problems or what made their immune system deficient in the first place may not even be Lyme related. Lyme and coinfections simply thrive in an environment that is compromised. As your immune system struggles to get Lyme under control, opportunistic infections can reactivate, such as herpes viruses and candida or yeast overgrowth.

Our bodies are a host for all sorts of microbes. When there is a burden, the balance is disrupted and our immune system is no longer able to keep those microbes in check. Think about how you can make it less of a breeding ground and make conditions unfavorable for bad microbes. Healing from Lyme could also be described as supporting the immune system and lessening the total burden of toxins and pathogens. Although intervention with antibiotics is helpful to bring down the pathogen load, ultimately the immune system must be able to contain the pathogens and take over at some point. Many people have rebalanced health, for example, by bringing down levels of glyphosate, aluminum, mold mycotoxins, parasites, and removing themselves from a toxic environment and only when the toxic load is low enough addressing Lyme and coinfection microbes.

In summary, Lyme microbes are not the only factor in the equation. They are often accompanied by other conditions that can add to the overall burden of your immune system which are described in the following sections.

MOLD

Mold and its toxic effects are not new. Mold was described in the Bible in the Old Testament where people were encouraged to burn their house if it was heavily affected by mold. After World War II, buildings were constructed increasingly sealed to conserve heat, yet this characteristic restricted the ability of a building to "breathe." Ritchie Shoemaker, a pioneer in the field of treatment for mold illness, estimates 50–70 percent of buildings have some kind of mold exposure. In today's modern environment, in rainy or coastal areas, mold is more often a problem than not (Shoemaker 2005). This context is important as 90 percent of our time is spent indoors breathing in air that's often more polluted than the air outdoors. Indoor air can be filled with mold spores, chemical gases, carpet fibers, dust, dander, bacteria, and dangerous viruses. You can be exposed to mold through food or the environment. Although in most cases, exposure is through the environment such as a moldy building, one should take measures to avoid continual exposure.

Mold deserves special treatment here due to its troublesome impact on people with Lyme. Indeed, Lyme and mold often go hand in hand. Many describe mold toxicity as the most common "comorbidity" or cofactor of Lyme and both have more recently been grouped together by some practitioners as "biotoxin illnesses." Mold and Lyme are both lipophilic toxins meaning that they are recirculated through the bile system and about a quarter of the population can't excrete these toxins properly due to genetics. Mold symptoms can mimic those of Lyme and can worsen symptoms in someone with Lyme. Long-chain fatty acids which are created by mold in the cell wall are also food for Lyme microbes.

There is a difference between growing mold which is living and mycotoxins which are the metabolized by-product of mold. Active growing mold is dealt with typically by antifungals and mycotoxins with binders. For many people with chronic Lyme, their immune systems are burdened and compromised so mold colonization is often a problem, meaning that the mold is living and growing inside them. In this case, antifungals, either pharmaceutical or herbal, should be considered.

At the very least, mold mycotoxins can suppress your immune function and, at the worst, make you very sick and cause more permanent illness triggering a condition called chronic inflammatory response syndrome (CIRS).

TESTING

Testing for mold is confusing and the recommendations from practitioners are varied. The following sections give a no-nonsense overview based on my trial and error and explain the difference in testing options so you can save money and get the most helpful results.

For the Human

To determine whether you have mold mycotoxins, there are urine tests by Great Plains Laboratory and RealTime Labs that will tell you if you've been exposed to mold and what types of mycotoxins you have. These two tests use different methodologies and will pick up different results, so using them together produces a better picture of the potential mold situation. Before doing a urine test, it is recommended to provoke excretion either by using a sauna or taking glutathione for several days before taking the sample. Organic Acid Test from Great Plains Laboratory can be helpful as there are metabolites that point to a possible mold problem. A urine test is helpful, but it is a moving target in that it indicates only what you are excreting. On the other hand, a mycotoxin antibody test like MyMycolab.com shows the antibody responses, indicating if the immune system is "at war" with the mycotoxins. A mycotoxin antibody test is useful as opposed to the urine tests, since it indicates whether the immune system is mounting a continual response which causes inflammation and symptoms.

There is also an online test called a visual contrast sensitivity test or VCS which can help determine if you are dealing with mold mycotoxins. The results reflect your overall toxic load and how your nervous system has been impacted. This test was developed by Dr. Shoemaker, who is a pioneer in the field. Shoemaker practitioners are those certified by the Shoemaker methodology and will measure other markers as well as genetic susceptibility to biotoxins. You can seek out a Shoemaker practitioner and refer to the website survivingmold.com for additional support.

For the House

The ERMI test, which stands for Environmental Relative Moldiness Index, analyzes the settled dust in buildings to determine the concentrations of DNA of the different mold species. ERMI scores range between –10 (good) and +20 (bad). Most people with CIRS with a high C4a cannot tolerate an ERMI score above +2. Another mold test is the HERTSMI, an acronym for Health Effects Roster of Type-Specific Formers of Mycotoxins and Inflammagens, which analyzes the dust sample provided for five mold species. The ERMI test screens for thirty-six mold species including the five from the HERTSMI. So the ERMI is more comprehensive and also includes mycotoxins testing which could reveal species not apparent from the HERTSMI. There are other options such as mold dishes. Companies like ImmunoLytics provide an analysis of cultured dishes which indicate the exact mold species. Although these dishes can help with remediation efforts, they are largely not as useful and less quantitative as the HERTSMI and ERMI scores. Both test kits can be ordered with the company Mycometrics. On top of these measures, a simple sniff test can also be helpful. If you sense a strong smell, which is created by the mold VOCs, you should do further testing. When making a significant decision to move, you should consult an experienced indoor environmental professional (IEP) in your area. An IEP is an experienced expert in building science and can do a thorough assessment of the area for the possibility of mold or other toxic exposure. To locate a certified IEP in your city, visit www.acac.org/find.

The readers are encouraged to order an ERMI test for where they are living as some people have gone through cycles of Lyme treatment unaware that they are affected by mold and see relief only when they remove themselves from a moldy environment.

WHAT TO DO

Finding a clean, mold-free environment should be the first on a checklist when going through treatment. Whether a person should treat mold or mold mycotoxins, as opposed to after the Lyme treatment, typically depends on how well they are managing their current detox load. Whether it takes priority over the Lyme treatment is a difficult decision to make and depends on the history of illness and onset of symptoms. Muscle testing may be useful to determine your main burden with the help of an experienced practitioner. Extreme mold avoidance, the concept of removing yourself from the exposure, can be helpful and may be warranted temporarily or for a longer period for more extreme cases. The book *A Beginner's Guide to Mold Avoidance* goes through more dramatic and practical measures to avoid mold exposure (Petrison and Johnson 2015).

The steps to deal with mold can be summarized as follows:

1) Remove yourself from the exposure by moving or remediating.

Based on the results from the tests mentioned above, you will have a better idea if mold is contributing to your symptom picture, and you might need to consider moving or remediation. Unfortunately, the bottom line is that if you are constantly in a moldy environment, your healing journey will be uphill, and you might not be able to get completely well. Also, when exposed to a moldy environment, unfortunately spores can cling to belongings, so when moving, this might mean leaving behind most clothes. Places that can be particularly problematic for mold are sinks, air-conditioning units, and washing machines. Cleaning of mold requires a special approach as a number of cleaners such as bleach could make the mold problem worse. Products from CitriSafe, such as the cleaners, sprays, and detergent, can be helpful.

2) Treat with antifungals to remove mold that is colonizing.

The immune system in a person with Lyme may not be able to keep mold colonization in check. So you may need to try different antifungals for several weeks to treat colonization in the GI tract, lungs, or sinuses, reviewing the dosage and potentially rotating antifungals with an experienced practitioner.

3) Helping the body remove the mycotoxins.

Mold mycotoxins can be removed with binders, such as clay, chlorella, and charcoal, among many other options. Which binders will be most helpful will depend on what mycotoxins are the biggest burden. For a list of binders that work for specific types of mold mycotoxins, refer to the book *Toxic* (Nathan 2018). When using binders, be mindful that they can pick up and move around toxins, so you might feel the effects of this movement.

It is important to consult your Lyme doctor before creating a plan, since these binders can also interfere with antibiotics and rob the body of precious fat-soluble vitamins. Also, detoxing mold can be too much of a burden for a person with Lyme already struggling to detox endotoxins or toxins that are created within the body from microbes and, at the very least, may require other liver support or opening up detox pathways as described later in this book.

Keep in mind that your LLMD may not be the right doctor to quarterback your mold detox plan, and you might need to seek out a specialist practitioner who can treat your mold. In some cases, LLMDs may even downplay the effects of mold. For more information on approaching mold, Dr. Jill Crista's book *Break the Mold* is a concise guide to treatment options, which use an herbal, nonpharmaceutical route (2018). There is much that can be done to prevent mold from becoming a problem over time with simple-to-implement measures, such as using a dehumidifier. For more information, Dr. Sandeep Gupta's online course summarizes mold illness and demystifies the concept around CIRS which many people with Lyme have trouble with.

AIR FILTERS

If your home has a high ERMI score, the options are remediation or moving as air filters are not a long-term solution to an ongoing mold problem. However, during the treatment process, you will have heightened sensitivity to mold or environmental contaminants, so a high-quality air filter should be a priority. Even after your Lyme journey, quality air filters are generally advisable as every day we breathe in over 15,000 L of air. They can be especially useful as a temporary solution when traveling or in between moves.

Even if you feel that mold is not a significant problem for you, as you go through your Lyme treatment, which could last from months to multiple years, you likely will have a mold exposure if you travel, move locations, or just in your day-to-day activities (or maybe you already are exposed in your home). You will be less able to deal with mold, compared to when you are not actively managing Lyme microbes. So by having heightened awareness and by using air filters, you will decrease any possible environmental toxins and have one less layer of the proverbial healing onion to unravel. Many people who have been in remission of symptoms from Lyme can experience a relapse when faced with a sudden mold exposure.

Mold reproduces by creating spores that vary in size, ranging from 2 to 100 microns. For comparison, a strand of human hair ranges from 17 to 181 microns in diameter. The following list describes the main residential filters currently on the market, which have been demonstrated in studies and independent laboratory tests to effectively clean and, in some cases, eliminate mold spores. These filters vary by price and square-foot coverage.

FILTER MODEL	TECHNOLOGY	UV
IQAir	Proprietary HyperHEPA filter to kill mold spores and filter out all the particles.	No
High Tech Air Solutions	Proprietary filters with UV-C lamps. The company sells larger units for installing in the home or a business.	Yes
Air Doctor Pro	Multiple layer filters including an UltraHEPA filter.	No
Molekule	Photo-electrochemical oxidation or PECO filter which uses reactive free radicals to break down pollutants including mold spores, bacteria, viruses, and other allergens (versions other than the mini are recommended for the option to disable the Wi-Fi function).	Yes
EnviroKlenz	UV air purifier that exposes the mold spores to the UV-C lights above the HEPA filter.	Yes
Hypoallergenic Air	Several proprietary technologies that replicate the ion balances of outdoor air to hinder growth of mold and pathogens both in the air and on surfaces.	Yes
Austin Air	Four-stage medical-grade HEPA filter and activated carbon.	No

Although not a filter, a propolis diffuser can be useful, along with ozone generators which can reduce the load of spores in a space (care must be taken to avoid breathing in the ozone and turning on the generators when the room is not occupied). For temporary situations, CitriSafe or EC3 products can be useful, as candles and dispensers that emit a safe, odorless concentrate that helps to reduce mold and balance the environment.

HEAVY METALS

Heavy metals can also impede the body's ability to heal as the body focuses on metabolizing the metals instead of fighting infections. High levels of aluminum are common with Lyme. Aluminum acts like fuel to Lyme, whereas mercury is the other culprit and can impair the immune system. Typical sources of mercury are seafood, amalgams (yours or your mother's), vaccines, or other implants.

To determine your levels of heavy metal toxicity, you can do both blood and urine tests (with Great Plains). Some metals come out better in urine, some in stool, some in hair. In terms of a hair analysis, an inch of hair closest to the skull represents exposure in the last four to six weeks. If it doesn't show toxicity of a particular metal, it doesn't mean it hasn't been a problem. Although slight elevations may indicate toxicity, a blood test is not generally indicative as metals stay in the blood for only short periods and then go into other areas. The body tries to maintain levels of minerals and metals constant in the blood and does this by moving them in and out of tissues. So blood levels are not telling you what's really stored in tissues, fat, and bone. Many metals including mercury are stored in tissues, especially in fats. If a urine heavy metals test is not provoked, meaning you are not forcing the release of metals, it will not be very helpful in showing the true heavy metal load in the body. So a more accurate test is a urine challenge test with DMSA or EDTA. The most accurate way to test heavy metal burden is by doing a urine test through a testing company called Doctor's Data and provoking excretion. This test is done at home and it needs to be done under the close guidance of an experienced practitioner. However, most people with Lyme will not be able to handle this test even under the guidance of an experienced practitioner, as their overall detox capacity may be limited. A DMSA test, for example, that will show mercury toxicity is not recommended for someone with impaired detox abilities. It is also controversial in that there is concern that the mercury could be redistributed throughout the body. Additionally, a urine test is limited for someone who does not excrete toxins well. Testing for heavy metals is also complicated if the burden of parasites is high, since parasites can harbor several times their weight in toxins including heavy metals. So if you have parasite issues, the heavy metal test results may not be accurate. Considering these challenges with urine and blood testing, another tool called the OligoScan which uses light spectrophotometry can be insightful. The OligoScan uses the principle that chemical compounds absorb, emit, or reflect light (electromagnetic radiation) at a certain range of wavelength to determine amounts of trace elements, minerals, and heavy metals throughout the body. An OligoScan is noninvasive and involves a device scanning your hand in less than a minute.

Unless heavy metal numbers are significant or there is a history of exposure such as significant dental amalgams, most practitioners will prioritize bringing down Lyme and coinfections first and then deal with heavy metals later.

GI HEALTH

For naturopathic doctors, all disease begins in the gut. It is estimated that we have 50 trillion–70 trillion human cells, which pale in comparison to the 1.4 quadrillion bacteria and 10 quadrillion fungi that make up part of our microbiome. After the Human Microbiome Project in 2007 by the National Institutes of Health, we have a deeper understanding of the complexity of the microbes living in us. We can appreciate the fact that the human body has more than ten times the number of microbial cells as it does human cells and that these microbes, although not fully understood, play a key role in our overall health. Although the gut is within the body, it faces outward, like the skin, with microbes living both within the body and on the surface. The microbiome is a layer coating the surface of the digestive tract, oral cavity, sinuses, vaginal canal in women, under fingernails, and on the surface of our skin, and these microbes have a role in vitamin and hormone production, mood regulation, cravings, immune regulation, and gene expression. Although the human gut is formed from early-life exposure to microbes, health status, genetics, and local environmental factors, there is much that one can do to maintain a healthy microbiome.

When taking antibiotics, you should take a good probiotic of over 50 billion live cultures. Each time you take an antibiotic, you should also take a probiotic an hour or two away from the antibiotic. However, to fully support the gut microbiome, it is not advisable to completely depend on probiotics alone. You should also incorporate a variety of probiotics from food into your diet, such as sauerkraut, kimchi, kefir, yogurt, or other fermented foods as well as prebiotic fibers. Pay attention to the sugar content in kombucha, though, as it can be too high. Also, many people with Lyme struggle with leaky gut, which is a condition where the gaps in the intestinal lining allow bacteria and other toxins to pass into the bloodstream, leading to additional inflammation. A shortcut to prevent and address leaky gut is through eliminating grains and legumes. Also helpful when dealing with leaky gut are foods that help repair the gut lining, such as bone broth collagen and aloe vera juice. For most cases, a paleo diet is advisable. However, you should stay away from foods that your body is reactive or sensitive to. Make sure to get enough fiber in your diet as this will not only nourish you, but it will also help your gut health. Although the exact number for the adequate amount of fiber to support gut health is not known, research shows that a greater variety of both soluble and insoluble fiber is optimal. Studies show that the microbiome develops well if you add one new vegetable per day, for a total of thirty-two vegetable varieties per month. A test called a GI Map by Diagnostic Solutions gives you a snapshot of the health of your gut and can indicate whether you have more harmful gut bacteria than good, otherwise called dysbiosis. This test can also tell you if you have specific parasites or leaky gut issues. Until you resolve dysbiosis, digestive enzymes during meals can be helpful as a dysbiotic intestinal ecology inhibits enzyme secretion from the small intestine and bile production from the stomach, pancreas, and liver. When you supplement with digestive enzymes, the food is better assimilated and nutrients are more readily available. Since these digestive organs are not as busy producing enzymes, they can focus more on detoxifying microbes and toxins and repairing tissue.

Indeed, good digestion and gut health give the liver a break, prevent and repair damage from antibiotics, and increase immune strength. A significant portion of your immune system is due to the gut which has many functions. The microbiome represents a huge part of detox function and can affect anything from mood to cognitive abilities. The gut and brain are connected via the vagus nerve and communicate back and forth. If one isn't happy, the other won't be either. Many nutrients and neurotransmitters are produced in the gut. For example, the gut produces 400 times the melatonin as your brain. So as you heal your gut, your overall need for supplements may decrease. Also, part of your healing will go hand in hand with gut health. In fact, by treating the microbes, your gut will be quicker to heal itself.

PARASITES

If you live in our modern society, you likely have parasites, especially if you eat meat, raw sushi, and raw vegetables without washing them properly, or have a dog. Some parasites are considered nonpathogenic and typically are not treated by conventional medicine. Parasites can also serve a useful role within our body such as sequestering toxins. However, with Lyme, these parasites can add to the overall immune system burden and also harbor Lyme spirochetes along with other bacteria. Parasites also suppress your innate immune system (and shift your immune system to a state called TH2 dominance).

For these reasons, many holistic practitioners opt to treat parasites before Lyme and coinfections. When treating parasites, keep in mind that since *Babesia* is a protozoa parasite and the same antimicrobials can have activity against *Babesia*. And vice versa, a *Babesia* protocol can have activity on parasites. Symptoms of parasites can be varied and include abnormal stool, irritability, hyperactivity, fatigue, symptom flare-ups around the full moon, pot belly, tummy aches, anal itching, visual acuity floaters, blurry vision, and food cravings.

In traditional cultures around the world, people take antiparasitic herbs preventatively and for maintenance. In modern society, we've largely lost these practices, such as accompanying our meals with spices and bitters. Although in some culinary cultures, such as with sushi, ginger and wasabi are still used. In Chinese medicine, a common recommendation is to eat primarily warm or hot food. Although this helps to support the spleen, another benefit of hot food is avoiding parasites and worms that could be introduced with raw food. When in treatment, you might take extra precautions as your system will already be working hard and less able to ward off new pathogens. Even with vegetables from the supermarket, it is recommended to properly clean them, for example with baking soda, HOCl, or vinegar prior to preparing them.

Unfortunately, in the Western world today, parasites are almost taboo and thought to only be problematic when traveling. However, parasites are everywhere and you don't need to go to a developing country to pick them up. There is also no bulletproof test for detecting all types of parasites as they can live in different organs and tissues outside of the intestinal tract. Stool tests such as the GI Map can show only the ones in your gut at best and in the sample. With the low accuracy using stool samples in many labs, parasitology research has not advanced compared to other microbe testing. Some parasites don't replicate and are not transmissible so will not be found even in the stool test. These parasites will use the body as a final host and impair the immune system. Genova Diagnostics and Meridian Valley Lab both specialize in testing for parasites. Practitioners proficient in muscle testing can also detect if parasites are significant stressors.

While killing parasites, be mindful that as parasites are flushed out, their toxins, such as ammonia, mold, heavy metals, or other neurotoxins, will be released as well. So a parasite cleanse should have binders on board. Activity of parasites follows the phases of the moon as levels of melatonin and serotonin in the body change, which then increases parasite activity. So parasite cleanses around the new moon and full moon can be particularly effective when repeated for several moon cycles or months.

Beyond the physical level, parasites can have a direct impact on our behavior and thoughts (Zimmer 2000). Many people struggling with parasites can relate to parasitic relationships described in the book *Dodging Energy Vampires* by Christiane Northrup, MD, and anecdotally comment that when they bring intention to their relationships, they experience healing progress (2018).

ADRENAL DYSFUNCTION

Proper adrenal function supports the immune function. Adrenal stress can be tested with simple saliva kits to test cortisol levels throughout the day. Keep in mind that while your body deals with illness, cortisol levels may not be within normal range, and as you recover, your adrenals will regain functionality. Over time with chronic stress, the adrenals try to help us survive in the best way they know how to. Adrenal hormones such as cortisol and DHEA are reduced as the adrenals try to keep up with the demand, stretched thin over time. When both these hormones are low, inflammation increases and dysregulation of blood sugar occurs. As a result, the person experiences symptoms of chronic fatigue, pain, weight around the middle, and irregular sleep patterns. Also, the adrenals manage the balance between sodium and potassium. Chronic infections deplete the body of electrolytes, making it more challenging to maintain normal hormonal and neurological function. So during recovery and treatment, electrolytes from trustworthy brands like Quinton to support adrenal fatigue can be very helpful.

YEAST

When treating Lyme you do not want yeast overgrowth as it

will impair your immune system and will make Lyme harder to treat. Yeast is a natural part of the gut flora, but it can get out of hand when the immune system is compromised with infection or toxic overload. Yeast is an insidious fungus that makes your body sluggish, and overgrowth can cause excess cytokine production and mimic many Lyme symptoms such as:

- Bloating, thrush, vaginal infections
- IBS, dysmenorrhea, endometriosis, bad breath, headaches
- Skin rashes, chronic sinus infections
- UTIs, ear pain, tinnitus
- Lymphatic swelling, joint pains, muscle pains
- Burning pains (skin and muscles)
- Red cheeks or ears, rosacea, white tongue
- Thin build or heavier set
- Overreaction to sugar
- Brain fog
- Fatigue
- Hashimoto's (elevated antibodies)
- An out-of-body "drunk-like" appearance

Yeast is treatable with herbal options, such as caprylic acid, oil of oregano, and garlic, along with prescription medications such as nystatin and Diflucan. In addition to antifungals, it is recommended to follow an anti-candida diet for several months. Yeast feeds off sugar and thrives in areas where the pH does not support growth of *Lactobacillus* and *Bifidobacterium* which are healthy bacterial strains that keep the growth of yeast in check. This anti-inflammatory elimination diet is not meant for prolonged use, although most practitioners recommend it for at least six months to see results. Many herbal tinctures and homeopathic remedies contain alcohol. So if you need to take these, the recommendation is to mix hot water with the tinctures so that the alcohol evaporates.

There is no cut-and-dry test for candida, but a good indicator is a protein called arabinose in the Organic Acids Test by Great Plains. If arabinose is high, it could indicate yeast, and you might want to consider treatment. As you treat Lyme, the immune system is better able to keep in check opportunistic infections such as candida.

DENTAL HEALTH

One of the most overlooked areas for some Lyme cases is dental health. We like to think of dental health as separate from our overall health. However, this thinking could not be more misguided. The nerves from our teeth are connected directly to the brain and each tooth has a connection to different organs and functions in a body. Also, our teeth are inches away from our brain and thyroid, so with any infection in a tooth or jaw, there is risk that it spreads to other areas. Biological dentistry seeks to treat dental health as part of overall health. As such, biological dentists use biocompatible materials which do not cause a significant toxic load to the body or create energetic disturbances.

In the 1950s, Fritz Kraemer, DDS, and Reinhold Voll, MD, determined that infected teeth can affect different organs in the body. Using an electro-acupuncture instrument, Dr. Kraemer found that each tooth correlates to an acupuncture meridian and to the meridian's corresponding organs and tissues.

TRADITIONAL CHINESE MERIDIAN ORGANS

Upper Teeth (1–16)

Heart, Small Int., Circulation/Sex, Triple Warmer
Right: Shoulder, elbow, hand (ulnar), sacroiliac joint, foot, toes, middle ear, right heart, right duodenum, terminal ileum, CNS, ant. pituitary

Stomach/Pancreas
Right: TMJ, anterior hip/knee, medial ankle
Sinus: Maxillary, oropharynx, larynx, esophagus, Right side of stomach
#2 parathyroid, #3 thyroid, right breast

Lung/Large Intestine
Right: Shoulder, elbow, hand (radial), foot, big toe
Sinus: Paranasal, ethmoid, bronchus, nose, right lung, right side of large intestine
#4 right breast

Liver/Gallbladder
Right: Post. hip/knee, lateral ankle
Sinus: Sphenoid, palatine tonsil, eye, hypothal., right liver, gallbladder

Kidney/Bladder
Right: Post. knee, sacroiliac joint, post. ankle
Sinus: Frontal pharyngeal tonsil, pineal, Right kidney, bladder, ovary, uterus, prostate, testicle, rectum

1	2	3	4	5	6	7	8
ASSOCIATED WESTERN MEDICINE JOINTS, ORGANS, AND GLANDS							
16	15	14	13	12	11	10	9

Heart, Small Int., Circulation/Sex, Triple Warmer
Left: Shoulder, elbow, hand (ulnar), sacroiliac joint, foot, toes, middle ear, left heart, jejunum, ileum, CNS, ant. pituitary

Stomach/Spleen
Left: TMJ, ant. hip/knee, medial ankle
Sinus: Maxillary, oropharynx, larynx, esophagus, left side of stomach
#14 thyroid, #15 parathyroid, left breast

Lung/Large Intestine
Left: Shoulder, elbow, hand (radial), foot, big toe
Sinus: Paranasal, ethmoid, bronchus, nose, left lung, left side of large intestine
#13 left breast

Liver/Biliary Ducts
Left: Post. knee, hip, lateral ankle
Sinus: Sphenoid, palatine tonsil, eye, hypothal., left liver, biliary ducts

Kidney/Bladder
Left: Post. knee, sacroiliac joint, post. ankle
Sinus: Frontal pharyngeal tonsil, pineal, left kidney, bladder, ovary, uterus, prostate, testicle, rectum

Lower Teeth (17–32)

Kidney / Bladder
Left: Post. knee, Sacroiliac joint, post. ankle
Sinus: Frontal pharyngeal tonsil, adrenal, left kidney, bladder, ovary, uterus, prostate, testicle, rectum

Liver/Gallbladder
Left: Post. hip/knee, lateral ankle.
Sinus: Sphenoid, palatine tonsil, eye, ovaries, testes. Ovaries, testes. Left liver, biliary ducts

Stomach/Spleen
Left: TMJ, ant. hip/knee, medial ankle
Sinus: Maxillary, oropharynx, larynx, esophagus, left side of stomach
#21: ovaries, testes, left breast

Lung/Large Intestine
Left: Shoulder, elbow, hand (radial), foot, big toe
Sinus: Paranasal, ethmoid, bronchus, nose, left lung, left side of large intestine

Heart, Small Int., Circulation/Sex, Triple Warmer
Left: Shoulder, elbow, hand (ulnar), sacroiliac foot, toes, middle ear, left heart, jejunum, ileum, CNS, ant. pituitary

24	23	22	21	20	19	18	17
ASSOCIATED WESTERN MEDICINE JOINTS, ORGANS, AND JOINTS							
25	26	27	28	29	30	31	32

Kidney / Bladder
Right: Post. knee, sacroiliac joint, post. ankle.
Sinus: Frontal pharyngeal tonsil, adrenal, right kidney, bladder, ovary, uterus, prostate, testicle, rectum

Liver/Gallbladder
Right: Post. hip/knee, lateral ankle.
Sinus: Sphenoid, palatine tonsil, eye, ovaries, testes, right, liver, gallbladder

Stomach/Pancreas
Right: TMJ, ant. hip/knee, medial ankle
Sinus: Maxillary, oropharynx, larynx, esophagus, right side of stomach
#28: ovaries, testes

Lung/Large Intestine
Right: Shoulder, elbow, hand (radial), foot, big toe
Sinus: Paranasal, ethmoid, bronchus, nose, right lung, right side of large intestine

Heart, Small Int., Circulation/Sex, Triple Warmer
Right: Shoulder, elbow, hand (ulnar), Sacroiliac joint, foot, toes, middle ear, right heart, right duodenum, terminal ileum, CNS

Dental infections, from root canals to cavitations, can also affect the vagus nerve which may have already been impaired by Lyme coinfections such as *Babesia*, and as a result, impair someone's detox ability as described later in this book.

Most dental issues fall into the following four categories.

CAVITATIONS

This area of "chronic ischemia" or lack of blood supply is referred to using various terms such as osteonecrosis, osteomyelitis, NICO, and so forth. It can also be described as a dental focal infection. The term *focal infection* implies that even though the source of the infection is in the mouth, the infection may be causing symptoms in other parts of the body, from the arm, thyroid, or even the heart. Sometimes these areas don't create symptoms. Removal of a focal infection should be performed by a trained biological dentist. Unfortunately, it's too common that when a tooth is removed, some of the periodontal ligament, which are the fibers that attach from the tooth to the gum and are prone to infection, can later reinfect this site. So when having a cavitation cleaned or a tooth extracted, the periodontal ligament needs to be completely removed. Part of a successful cavitation surgery may include L-PRF (leukocyte- and platelet-rich fibrin) which is made from one's blood, ozone to clean out the area, lasers for speeding up the healing and managing symptoms, avoiding the use of vasoconstrictors such as steroids, and isopathic remedies such as AsperSAN and NotaSAN, which many people opt to use in place of systemic antibiotics.

ROOT CANALS

There are approximately 20 million root canal procedures per-formed each year in the United States alone which represents a large industry, so questioning their existence is controversial at best. Each tooth is an organ with blood and nerve supply. Performing a root canal kills the tooth. So you are leaving a dead organ in your mouth, which becomes a hotel for all sorts of anaerobic microbes and parasites. In a root canal site, dead tissue remains in microscopic canals and becomes an additional burden for your immune system. In conventional dentistry, it is believed that the site is completely cleaned. However, physicians are realizing that in practice, this is not the case.

A study published by the American Academy of Periodontology found that in half of the subjects studied, the root-canaled tooth and the patient's blood contained bacteria tracing back to the original site of infection (Debelian et al. 1998). Also in conventional dentistry, the toxic Gutta-percha compound is used, which overflows into the roots and nerve matrix and then drains into the rest of the body. Due to the popular *Root Cause* documentary and books such as the *Root Canal Cover-Up*, there is more awareness around the possible long-term negative consequences of root canals (Bailey 2019; Meinig 2008). Physicians who are leaders in their field are beginning to put together the pieces. For example, Dr. Thomas Rau, director of the cancer prevention clinic Paracelsus in Switzerland, noted that of 150 of his breast cancer patients, 147 of these patients had one or more root canals in the same meridian as the original cancer tumor. Also, some savvy cardiologists are known to recommend removal of infected teeth much before a patient undergoes heart surgery.

In the case of people with Lyme, root canals can act as a reservoir for Lyme and coinfections and also other pathogenic bacteria. For example, here is a lab result from my root canal tooth (using a lab called DNA Connections) showing multiple Lyme microbes after a year of antibiotic and other therapeutic interventions.

TEST RESULTS

Sample type: **#18 Root Canal Tooth**

This test utilizes polymerase chain reaction technology to detect the presence of targeted microbial DNA for the causative agent of Lyme disease and common tick-transmitted coinfections. Sensitivity of the test is 1 to 10 microbes with a specificity exceeding 5x10.

The ✓highlighted microbes were detected in the submitted sample:

Borrelia burgdorferi F7

✓B. burgdorferi Osp A-IND

B. burgdorferi Osp B

B. burgdorferi Osp C

Babesia microti

✓Babesia divergens-IND

✓Babesia duncani-NPS

Bartonella bacilliformis

✓Bartonella henselae-NPS

Bartonella quintana

✓Borrelia miyamotoi-IND

Borrelia recurrentis

Ehrlichia chaffeensis

Anaplasma phagocytophilium

NONE

If the tooth is not removed, these pathogens stay in the site and can drain into the rest of the body, complicating treatment and staying as a burden to the immune system. Savvy biological dentists observe that some people only truly respond to treatment when they get their root canals or other dental focal infections taken care of. Removal of root-canaled teeth should follow the principles described above as part of a cavitation surgery (L-PRF, laser therapy, ozone water and gas, avoiding vasoconstrictors, use of AsperSAN and NotaSAN or other homeopathy remedies). When planning any surgery, it is recommended to work with your LLMD and consider having antimicrobials on board since some infection will be released during the procedure.

AMALGAMS

When you have different metals in your mouth, a current is created and generates an electromagnetic disturbance. Incompatible dental fillings can also be damaging and generate inflammation. Dental materials and fillings can contain BPA which is a carcinogen. Even a dental structure that appears relatively innocuous, a stainless steel band for example, can leach nickel and iron into your body over time. Mercury fillings slowly leach into your mouth over time with chewing and drinking hot liquids. The mercury is then stored throughout your body, especially fatty tissues like the brain. Mercury fillings must be removed by an experienced and qualified dentist. Not doing so and not having an appropriate detox plan during removal can cause much harm.

MALOCCLUSION

Structural problems with the jaw or a misaligned bite can cause all sorts of repercussions for your body's ability to detox and the proper functioning of the autonomic nervous system. A poor bite can have a cascade of downstream effects that impact your overall health, described at length in the book *Breath* by James Nestor (2020).

WHAT TO DO

This section only scratches the surface on the main considerations with regard to oral and dental health which may or may not play a significant role in your situation. If you believe this topic is affecting your health—for example, if you started to feel worse or more symptomatic around the time of a dental intervention—then you might want to pay more attention to this topic or dig a little deeper.

Biological Dentist

The quality of biological dentists varies on a spectrum and you might need to research before settling on one. Unfortunately, there is no objective criteria or regulatory institution for qualifying a dentist as holistic or biological. Once you find a good biological dentist, start working with them on all the possible dental health issues. You might need to travel to see them and pay a premium including additional cone beam CT scans or workups that aren't covered with traditional dentistry or insurance. For guidance on stealth "focal" infections and proper dental health, Dr. Louisa Williams has done extensive work in the area combining her experience in homeopathy and other energetic modalities and published the book *Radical*

Medicine. Dr. Williams also explains a protocol for cavitation surgery and amalgam removal (2011).

Bioelectric Testing

An acupuncture meridian assessment (AMA) uses a fixed 2.4 V circuit where your body, or more specifically your body's energy meridians, are the resistor in the circuit. It's hard to find practitioners, but you can search online for those in your area. This technique can be extremely useful not just for dental scans but whole-body scans to find out which organ systems are stressed.

Cone Beam Scan

Stealth dental infections don't usually show up until they are more advanced. With X-rays, 30–50 percent of bone must be destroyed before signs of alarm become evident. However, that is a negative X-ray, when no clear radiolucency or black hole is apparent, but it does not necessarily signify there is no infection. Instead, it's necessary to get a cone beam X-ray. Apart from detecting dental health issues, calcification of the pineal gland can also be observed. In addition to the cone beam scan, a thermography which shows increased heat can be helpful in indicating possible infections.

Oral Health Routine

You can strengthen and remineralize your teeth, even reverse early cavities, through cell salts, silica, Quinton electrolytes, a good dental hygiene routine, and the right diet based on Weston A. Price and described in the section below. Massaging organs and lymph that infected teeth may be affecting such as the thyroid can be helpful. Maintain the right pH in your mouth. Unfortunately, many people drink a lot of lemon water to alkalize the body which can erode teeth enamel when done frequently over time. To avoid this, rebalance saliva pH by gargling with warm salt (and baking soda) water. Be proactive and have good dental hygiene practices and check your nutrition for fat-soluble vitamins and minerals to remineralize teeth, oil pull, and so on. Don't let problems drag on. Dental health plays a significant role in overall health.

Oil Pulling

This technique is helpful for chelating fat-soluble toxins. A big mouthful of organic coconut or sesame oil is held in the mouth for as long as possible, usually three to ten minutes and then spit out. During this time, these toxins in the oral mucosa as well as circulating in the blood vessels traveling through the oral mucosa are absorbed into the oil. This therapy helps absorb toxic chemicals traveling in the blood from other parts of the body as they are passing through. After spitting out the oil (making sure not to swallow any of it), gargle with salt and baking soda and then brush your teeth. You can do this practice once or twice a day.

Dental Diet

The Canadian dentist Weston A. Price pioneered a way of thinking about nutrition for oral and dental health in the 1930s. From his work studying traditional societies around the globe in fourteen different countries, he concluded that the societies that had the greatest longevity, healthy jaw structure, and almost no cavities had a nutrient-dense diet in common that consisted of foods rich in fat-soluble vitamins A, D, and K2. Since Weston A. Price, additional work has been published that reinforce his findings. *The Dental Diet* by Steven Lin outlines a modern approach to obtaining these nutrients and explains recent science that supports the recommendations (2018). Also, the recipe book *Nourishing Traditions* by Sally Fallon describes at length recipes that include traditional fats (clean animal fats, cod liver oil, dairy fats, olive oil), organic fruits and vegetables, raw dairy products, soured or fermented dairy and vegetables like sauerkraut and kimchi, whole grains (soaked or soured to neutralize phytic acid and lectins), and bone stocks (1999).

Of all the factors that can affect one's healing journey, dental and oral health may be the most pernicious and stealthy of them all. Due to the mobility of Lyme and coinfections and their affinity for hiding in dead tissue, your mouth may be negatively contributing to your overall health. You might not respond adequately to treatment protocols until you address your dental and oral health issues. Whether this is the case depends on your situation. The reader is encouraged to seek out a biological dentist and additional support if there are concerns based on past dental history.

VIRUSES

Many viruses can be transmitted within a tick or other insect bites and are often not accounted for in treatment protocols. Indeed, many of these viruses don't even have names and are often overlooked by doctors focusing on the bacteria *Borrelia*. However, these viruses require very different treatment protocols. In fact, it is also thought by some practitioners that rotation of long-term antibiotics is effective as several antibiotics have antiviral activity. Recent work on retroviruses by Kent Heckenlively and researcher Judy Mikovits, PhD, in their book *Plague: One Scientist's Intrepid Search for the Truth about Human Retroviruses and Chronic Fatigue Syndrome (ME/CFS), Autism, and Other Diseases* sheds more light on this topic which hasn't been well understood and plays an important role in Lyme Disease (2014). The other viruses commonly seen are opportunistic ones, such as EBV, CMV, and HPV6, that become active when the immune system is overburdened. As Lyme is dealt with and the immune system comes back into balance, these viruses often are less problematic.

NUTRITIONAL DEFICIENCIES

Your diet should aim to provide for your body's nutrients; however, dealing with microbes can deplete nutrients and you will likely need to supplement. There are many labs to check nutritional deficiencies including NutrEval or SpectraCell. There is also a scan called an OligoScan which takes thirty seconds and gives you an overall snapshot of nutrient deficiencies as well as toxicity level. Many people with Lyme are deficient in magnesium, B6, vitamin D, zinc, B12, folate, copper, and sometimes trace minerals such as chromium and most can also benefit from supplementing with whole food iodine and selenium to support the thyroid. Deficiencies can result in muscle pains and cramps, poor concentration, poor metabolic health, adrenal fatigue, cravings, and anxiety, among many other symptoms. Since the process of treating and recovering can deplete nutrients, it is advisable to use a good-quality multivitamin at some point. People also do well on a healthy dosage of vitamin D, checking levels periodically.

Choose your multivitamin wisely, as some multivitamins can cause reactions due to fillers or binders; work up low and slow to the recommended dosage.

Although there is limited literature on the subject, there is a condition called kryptopyrroluria (KPU) where a by-product of hemoglobin synthesis is elevated in the urine. Since HPLs bind to zinc, biotin, manganese, vitamin B6, and other important compounds, the body becomes depleted in these substances. Regarding Lyme and chronic illness, Dr. Klinghardt has found the incidence of KPU in Lyme Disease to be 80 percent or higher and believes it may be an inherited condition or possibly induced by chronic infections. When KPU is an issue, there are numerous negative implications for the immune system and detoxification. To address the condition, a multivitamin and mineral supplement like Core S from Biopure is recommended, along with supporting copper levels. For more information on testing, readers are recommended to review the article "Kryptopyrroluria (aka Hemopyrrollactamuria): A Major Piece of the Puzzle in Overcoming Chronic Lyme Disease" by Scott Forsgren (2009).

HYPERCOAGULABILITY

Although one may not have heard of the term *hypercoagulability*, one may be dealing with it on a recurring basis. Viruses, bacteria, and mold can all lead to an inflammatory state which triggers increased coagulation and results in the formation of an insoluble mesh-like protein called fibrin. The signs and symptoms associated with hypercoagulability are related to diminished blood flow, such as light-headedness, dysautonomia, and postural tachycardia syndrome (POTS). To help ease the symptoms of hypercoagulability, many doctors may recommend blood thinners throughout the process of Lyme treatment which may include proteolytic enzymes like lumbrokinase, serrapeptase, and nattokinase. These enzymes are often recommended since they reduce inflammation, can potentiate other antibiotics, and break up biofilms. Although you may experience benefits and reduced related symptoms in taking these enzymes, to address hypercoagulability, the root cause should ultimately be addressed. As you address the most problematic pathogens, such as viral and bacterial infections, the hypercoagulability should resolve.

6

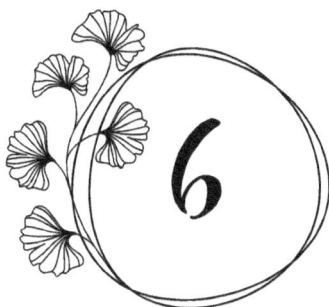

SUPPORTIVE AND ALTERNATIVE THERAPIES

As alluded to in previous chapters, antibiotic therapy is not a panacea. Fortunately, there are other options. If someone with Lyme follows the standard of care, which at the time of writing is antibiotic protocols with LLMDs, and still doesn't get relief or gets only some level of relief, they must look elsewhere for solutions out of necessity. Although some of the following modalities are not accepted, or are even ridiculed, in Western medicine the person still suffering with symptoms opts to try them since the benefit and possibility to regain health outweighs the risk.

The following list is a summary of some of the most effective options, which are listed in the registry for MyLymeData.org. Some therapies are meant to be supporting or adjunct—in other words, not a primary or stand-alone therapy—whereas other therapies have offered some complete remission and have been used as a stand-alone modality with much success. Many of these therapies can be combined and done in parallel. The following section overviews the main therapies and discusses their associated best practices or tips.

ACUPUNCTURE

A one-off acupuncture session cannot be expected to have a tremendous impact. Rather, an ongoing commitment of several months, normally once or twice a week, is required. Acupuncture is based on energy meridians and has been practiced for hundreds of years in Chinese medicine. Finding a good practitioner ideally with experience in Lyme Disease treatment is key. It can help organs function better, boost immune function, help sleep, detox functions, among many benefits and alleviates symptoms more generally, which is a significant part of the battle. Especially when you are going through cleansing or treatments, regular acupuncture can prevent blockages or imbalances in your body to detox properly. Acupuncture helps correct a number of issues from Bell's palsy to helping to heal damaged tissues.

OZONE

Ozone, although not currently supported by the FDA in the United States, is used in many other parts of the world for a variety of use cases. Ozone can be administered in different ways depending on where the target ailment is or what organs you are looking to affect. To use ozone intravenously, it is important to work with experienced and trained practitioners as there are risks involved. One should work up to the dosage of gamma, a measure for ozone concentration, along with the amount of blood treated. Typically, treatments can be twice a week for several weeks until symptom relief. Using ozone intravenously, it can stimulate the immune system by as much as 400 percent to produce the cytokine molecules that the body uses to fight infections and can promote TH1 immune function, which many people dealing with chronic infection obtain much benefit from. Apart from intravenous, many people find benefit in rectal or intestinal insufflation, using multiple treatments per week over multiple months. Some people find so much benefit that many invest in a professional ozone generator from companies such as Longevity Resources or Simply O3. Anecdotally, many people experience tremendous healing with frequent and repeated use of rectal or intestinal ozone. Many comment that this might be the most effective and safe therapy that one can do from home. Apart from the initial machine investment, which will be around a $1,000, the costs are $20 to pick up an industrial oxygen tank at Home Depot, for example, which will last four to six months.

Many people think the benefit of ozone comes from killing pathogens. However, a more beneficial impact is the improvement of oxygen delivery to your cells. Immune cells convert oxygen into ozone, hydrogen peroxide, and free radicals to destroy pathogens. Anything that increases the oxygen that reaches those cells makes them more effective. People may also comment that ozone makes them feel "normal"—that is, asymptomatic. This reminder in and of itself, however, may be considered a win and worth the treatment. However, symptoms creep back after the effects of treatment wear off. The book *Ozone Miracle* goes into detail about the uses, specifically how to use this therapy in a safe manner from the comfort of one's home (Shallenberger 2017).

FASTING

Humans are one of the few mammals who don't go into the forest and fast when they are sick. Fasting can have tremendous benefits and can reset your gut microbiome and immune system (Buhner 2012). Indeed, there have been many accounts of people with Lyme fasting for several days on end, such as seven-to-ten-day fasts multiple times a year and significantly improving their symptoms or experiencing remission. Even two-to-three-day fasts can be significant for resetting gut bacteria. Your intestinal lining completely regenerates itself in three days. Fasting can also be effective for parasite cleanses around the moon cycles. However, multiple-day fasts should ideally be done with close professional guidance, review of blood work, monitoring of electrolyte levels and symptoms. It is advisable that you seek professional help and work with a doctor if you are planning a longer fast. For example, specialized clinics such as True North in California can help guide you and monitor you onsite throughout a fast. Fasting also helps support the liver as it will be free of other tasks, such as breaking down food and processing nutrients. Indeed, a liver cleanse, which can be a form of a fast, avoids fats and animal proteins that put more of a strain on the liver. Unfortunately, antibiotics and supplements need to be taken with food or fats, which makes multiple-day fasts unfeasible. However, you can try an overnight fast of sixteen hours where you eat breakfast later in the day and avoid eating four hours before bed. For those who find water fasting is not an option or for those who don't have a doctor to monitor the process, a fasting-mimicking diet, consisting of a plant-based diet primarily of vegetables and minimal protein and fats, can produce some of the effects of fasting.

Additionally, limiting the eating window to six to eight hours can be beneficial, otherwise known as intermittent fasting, with the first meal at 11:00 a.m. and the last meal at 6:00 p.m. If you're tired of tracking, a fasting app called Zero helps with tracking. In terms of timing a fast, be mindful of stressful periods, as fasting in and of itself is a stress on the body. Listen to your body if intermittent fasting doesn't feel right or slows down your metabolism. It might not be right for you, or you might need to do it less frequently.

HYDROTHERAPY AND COLD EXPOSURE

Popularized by the Wim Hof method, exposure to cold temperatures has several benefits. When exposed to the cold, our body dilates and constricts blood vessels to manage our temperature. This movement of blood spreads around our immune cells. Cold therapy also activates your innate immune system. This is the one responsible for fighting Lyme. It is advisable to build up gradually using cold exposure. To begin, you can use cold temperatures at the end of a shower and then graduate to full ice baths. Dipping in an ice-cold bath of zero degrees for two minutes has significant anti-inflammatory effects that last several days. Also, it is important not to stay in cold water too long and to warm up your body after. The Wim Hof method recommends the horse stance, a posture and movement for generating heat and warming up your body. Not doing some activity to warm up your body, such as the horse stance or staying in the cold water too long, can make you sick. Doing this practice on a recurring basis every few days or even every day can have cumulative and a transformative impact in terms of reducing inflammation which will help with symptom relief (Carney 2017). There is a reason why people are called ice junkies because the feeling is almost addictive. Cold exposure also helps your central nervous system and trains your vagus nerve, which activates the parasympathetic branch of your autonomic nervous system and controls heart rate variability (HRV). Ice baths, cold showers, or swimming in a cold lake even on a recurring basis can have a dramatic positive impact on increasing HRV levels, which is a proven indicator of health according to multiple studies.

Once you are out of the ice-cold water, you can let your own body warm itself up as opposed to jumping in a hot shower. On the other hand, using contrast therapy when showering (changing from hot and cold) is helpful for immune function and increases mitochondria function. You don't have to jump in an ice bath, but you can turn up the coldest water for a minute and slowly work up to two minutes. There is a protocol for contrast therapy which consists of three minutes in the shower with hot water, followed by one minute of cold water, then alternating again with hot water for three minutes. and then again one minute of cold water. At the time of writing, a double-blind, controlled study was underway to quantify the effects of contrast hydrotherapy on the innate immune system of COVID patients (Ramirez et al. 2021). Throughout history and in different cultures, some form of contrast therapy was used. For example, during the Spanish flu before therapeutic interventions were available, people used a version of contrast hydrotherapy upon developing symptoms. The Finnish saunas provide another example. A Finnish study of sauna use five days a week found an overall 40 percent reduction in mortality from all causes (Laukkanen 2015).

An additional benefit of cold exposure is the reduction of inflammation. Part of your job when healing from Lyme is to bring down inflammation, as this will help you manage symptoms better. One way to do this is through a simple ice bath. The anti-inflammatory effects of a cold plunge in 32°F water between two and three minutes can last up to six days. So pace yourself; you can cold plunge every few days. If the water is not as cold, simply stay in longer. Some people benefit so much from the decrease in inflammation that they incorporate a cold plunge into their routine and invest in bathtub products, such as Morozko, Furo, and the Cold Plunge.

BIOENERGETIC

"If you want to find the secrets of the universe, think in terms of energy, frequency, and vibration."

—NIKOLA TESLA

For thousands of years, healers have understood that our health depends on the quality of energy that flows through us and makes up our bodies. Science has verified this insight through years of research and discoveries. However, the Western medicine paradigm was developed in the backdrop of the pharmaceutical industry, and many effective energetic therapies today are not mainstream or have not been commercialized.

Even though the conventional medical systems primarily see medicine through the lens of biochemistry, humans are bioelectromagnetic beings. The heart has an electrical system that coordinates the beating of different chambers so that blood flows to where it's needed around the body. We measure that electrical activity with an electrocardiogram (EKG). Similarly, the brain radiates brain waves constantly that we measure with an electroencephalogram (EEG). Organs generate electrical currents which then flow through tissues and in turn also generate magnetic fields through Ampère's law in and around the body. That's why magnetic field therapy works because it can stimulate these currents (Tennant 2014). Every living organism has a different frequency, a unit of measurement of a cycle of energy through time. When you are open to these concepts and begin to think of health from a lens of bioenergy, as opposed to biochemistry, a whole world of new tools and therapies start to emerge. Some people who have not seen significant progress with antibiotics have found relief and even full remission in bioenergetic therapies.

Others regret not incorporating bioenergetics from the start for support throughout treatment, from muscle testing of medications and supplements, acupuncture meridian assessment (AMA) to find imbalances in organs, checking food sensitivities, to innovative therapies like LymeStop. Sometimes what the body needs is less—less supplements and less antimicrobials. In an effort to manage daily life and out of desperation to get better, many people end up taking an abundance of supplements (and later accumulate a supplement graveyard) which can be taxing for the liver and the body's elimination systems. Interventions that make use of energetic therapies and support the immune system can be useful for these cases. The difference of opinion even between the most experienced practitioners on treatment plans can lead to frustration, economic burden, and lack of progress. Bioenergetic therapies, for example muscle testing, can help tease out the biggest stressors and determine the priorities of treatment plans. Unlike many therapies from antibiotics to supplements, which can be limited by access to what is in the bloodstream, the effects of bioenergetic therapies can penetrate more easily throughout the whole body, through organs, the blood-brain barrier, and into cells. After much work in functional medicine and detox, now-retired Dr. Neil Nathan goes into detail on the applications of energetic therapies in his latest book, *Energetic Diagnosis: Groundbreaking Thesis on Diagnosing Disease and Chronic Illness*, recommended reading for the reader interested in digging deeper into these tools (2022).

Wherever you are in your openness to incorporating these energetic modalities, the following is an overview of a few options chosen by popularity for supporting people with Lyme and coinfections.

FSM

FSM devices emit low levels of current set at specific frequencies which are determined based on a wide range of symptoms and medical problems. Microcurrent delivers a microamperage current—that is, 1,000 times less than milliampere current which is barely perceivable. The treatment is typically given through electrodes placed on your skin. FSM devices are FDA approved (as a TENS unit) for wound healing, pain control, and aesthetics. The treatment is low risk and side effects typically pass after the treatment. The correct frequencies are determined by an experienced practitioner and by observation of how the body responds to them. There are frequencies meant to address over 200 conditions from common conditions like inflammation, toxicity, muscle pain, or mineral deposits, to more specific conditions like polio virus and congestion. FSM is especially effective at treating nerve and muscle pain, inflammation, and scar tissue. It is different from other modalities described in the following sections. For example, FSM is different from Rife therapy, which is aimed at killing microbes, not treating inflammation or pain. It is also different from pulsed electromagnetic field (PEMF) as the latter operates at a higher voltage and is not specific for different conditions. Research has yet to be done to document each frequency's effects, and these protocols are meant to suggest efficacy and act as a guide. For example, studies on a specific microcurrent protocol showed increased ATP production by more than 400 percent, increased protein generation by 70 percent, and increased amino acid transport by 40 percent (McMakin 2017). Many of the studies on FSM have been spearheaded by Dr. Carolyn McMakin who pioneered work in the early 1990s and continues to train many practitioners. Like many modalities discussed in this section, one should seek the help of an experienced practitioner to guide treatment.

RIFE

In the 1950s, Dr. Royal Rife, an American doctor and inventor, created a machine that he claimed was capable of destroying pathogens. Dr. Rife believed that all diseases had a vibration, and if you could attack that disease with sound waves at a slightly higher vibration, the disease would be destroyed. This concept is essentially how the Rife machine works, with an amplifier, a frequency generator, a capacitor box, and a wire coil. It emits low electromagnetic waves that alter individual pathogens, applied through contact with the hands or feet. The premise is that all medical conditions have an electromagnetic frequency, and this machine will deliver pulses at the same frequency to disable diseased cells. Rife machines and other at-home electromagnetic frequency devices are not likely to cause any long-term risks, although no long-term randomized clinical trials have been done. The electromagnetic frequency they emit is very weak, sometimes too weak to even penetrate the skin. Modern Rife machines have preprogrammed options for Lyme which start first with an overall terrain or detox and later frequencies that target and kill specific microbes. Working with a skilled practitioner who can test you energetically via muscle testing, EAV, or other techniques is helpful, since the transmission of the frequencies is only as good as knowing which frequency to apply. Although many Rife machines are available to buy, this problem, determining which frequencies are needed, is why many people do not get far in using Rife technologies. Modern Rife technology incorporates biofeedback to assess which frequencies would be most needed by your body.

A newer, more affordable Rife machine called the Spooky2 has emerged in recent years to address these hurdles with a device that is accessible to the average consumer at a lower price tag. The Spooky2 has three modes of transmission: through contact where your hands hold the electrodes, through radio waves transmitted via an amplifier, through a tube or antenna, or via remote transmission. Anyone can download the Spooky2 software, but then they must buy a frequency generator. There is an infrared biofeedback system called Spooky2 Pulse that scans the body to detect all pathogens, pollutants, and parasites present, which helps to understand which frequencies of the 40,000 options in the database to use. Although Spooky2 is a powerful tool, there is a learning curve with using and configuring it. Other Rife technologies, such as True Rife and Resonant Light, exist at a higher price tag, and additional devices that make use of healing frequencies have emerged, such as the Healy device to simplify this technology for the average consumer.

HOMEOPATHY

Around 200 years ago, Dr. Samuel Hahnemann, the father of homeopathy, proposed the law of similars, that "like cures like" and healing effects happen by giving a small dose of a substance that causes those same symptoms in larger doses. Today, homeopathic concepts can be found in modern medicine in immunotherapy, for example. Homeopathic dilutions use very low concentrations that may even lack a molecule of the diluted physical substance, which can be either mineral, plant, medication, animal, or microbe. Although it may sound like at such high dilutions, the remedy would not be useful, the energetic imprint of the substance remains in the liquid dilution or the pellets and primarily change the water, which is the majority of what we are made out of. Readers interested in learning more about this area are encouraged to check out the book *The Hidden Messages in Water* by Masaru Emoto (2011). Homeopathy remedies can be used to treat acute issues, for managing symptoms, organ support, promoting lymph drainage, sleep, pain, and stress management. Some homeopathic remedies such as those from the brand Byron White can be used against specific microbes and coinfections. A homeopathic remedy called Nosodes are made from dead microbes, which provide the body with information to manage the symptoms created by the microbe. Apart from acute use cases, there is another field called *constitutional homeopathy* which aims to support an individual long term in a more holistic way with a single remedy that is personalized to what the person may need. This approach is based on miasms which are a grouping of constitutions, temperaments, physical characteristics, and family patterns, among other things that are tendencies within a person and create predisposition to disease. Homeopathy is also distinct from other therapies as it affects the physical body as well as the mental and emotional body.

Homeopathy receives much skepticism in the Western world and has not been adopted in the United States compared to other parts of the world like in Germany or Cuba, for example. Those who come to constitutional homeopathy have typically tried many other therapies and worked with many practitioners before with little success. Despite the decreasing number of homeopathic schools across the world, this system of medicine has stood the test of time as people who use homeopathy can attest to its impact. To learn more about constitutional homeopathy, readers are encouraged to review books published by both Dr. Divya Chhabra and Dr. Rajan Sankaran, who are the founders of the practice.

SOUND THERAPY

Sound therapy has been used in different periods in history around the world. There are sound chambers with frequencies imprinted in them in pyramids, for example, where people used to go for healing frequencies. Yoga mantras thousands of years in Sanskrit were used for therapeutic benefit. The advantage of sound therapy is that the effects can permeate more completely into the body, through the blood-brain barrier, unlike other applications that may reach a more superficial level. In terms of modern technologies, the AmpCoil and Sentient Element are two consumer devices that make use of sound healing. The AmpCoil and Sentient Element use sound frequencies delivered via a pulsed electromagnetic field (PEMF) to help get your cells back in "tune" and resonate with certain natural frequencies. Everything in the body from cells, tissues, to organs resonates at a certain frequency. Not unlike how a tuning fork works, by resonating a specific frequency these cells, tissues, and organs can get back into harmony and resume optimal function. The bioresonance coil is placed on the body, and a tablet that contains a software program prompts the coil to pulsate at specific frequencies. A recording of your voice with the tablet allows the software program to personalize the electromagnetic frequencies to address health deficits based on what the body needs. These frequencies then vibrate through the coil into your body and cells to boost many functions from blood flow, oxygen, nutrient transportation, to detoxification. The voice recording biofeedback option takes the guesswork out of deciding which frequencies to use, and the frequencies are all preprogrammed. Finally, the AmpCoil or Sentient Element works to rebalance the pH, which in effect creates a less favorable environment for yeast, parasites, and other pathogens.

LIGHT THERAPY

In photodynamic therapy, low-level or low-power lasers that cannot damage tissue in the body are used to apply light at certain frequencies to generate therapeutic effects. These effects can be cellular regeneration or can have activity against bacteria, parasites, and viruses. There are four different laser colors and different frequencies in which the treatments can be administered:

- **Red:** Promotes an increase in blood flow and a reduction in overall blood pressure.
- **Blue:** Anti-aging and anti-inflammatory effects, along with improving your cognitive ability.
- **Yellow:** Boosts mood and reduces the effects of other mood challenges by increasing your body's natural secretion of serotonin. The yellow laser also reduces the severity of chronic stress and helps the absorption of vitamin D.
- **Green:** Promotes metabolism, tissue repair, and skin hydration.

Among the many light- and photon-based therapies, a few stand out: the Weber laser, FREmedica device, and the Bionic 880 laser. FREmedica is a wearable frequency emitter specifically designed to manage chronic Lyme and its associated symptoms. There are different settings with the FREmedica device, with different goals from detox, balance, anxiety, and stress, to Lyme basic settings. Before-and-after impact can be assessed with an EAV device to determine the balance/stress of organ and meridian systems, or with muscle testing to determine signs of ongoing microbial stress. Unlike the FREmedica device which is focused on Lyme and coinfections, the Weber laser can be widely applied more broadly to other pathogens, such as viruses and parasites. At the time of writing, a study was underway that treats patients with COVID-19, for example. The treatment can be administered intravenously, interstitially, intra-articularly, transcranially, and externally (Weber et al. 2020). For intravenous use, it is important to work with an experienced practitioner. There is also a laser watch that applies light to the wrist arteries, with an applicator for the nose and mouth where a person can apply the treatment at home. Using a photosensitizer to capture the light, such as curcumin, riboflavin, and chlorophyll, the effect can kill pathogens using blue and UV light. Although there is limited clinical data with Lyme Disease, the anecdotal results look promising. For more information on the science, the International Society for Medical Applications (ISLA) was founded in Germany in 2005 as a research organization to study low-level laser therapy and has published many peer-reviewed clinical studies. Another biophoton device called the Bionic 880 has been used in Europe to treat *Borrelia* and coinfections, although it is not yet widely adopted in the United States or accepted by the FDA. It uses homeopathic remedies or nosodes. Several practitioners, such as Dr. Ingo Woitzel in Germany, claim a 90 percent success rate after several sessions. Another application of light therapy, not aimed at killing microbes directly, is using red and infrared light for supporting mitochondrial health. Many people with Lyme notice an immediate boost in energy using red and infrared light therapy along with decreased inflammation and improved sleep.

MAGNETIC THERAPY

A novel therapy called LymeStop uses magnets applied to certain points on the body to activate the neuroimmune system and creates a recognition of different microbes. Each pathogen from parasites, viruses, yeast, to *Borrelia* and coinfections corresponds to a different point on the body. The presence of the pathogen, or more precisely its stress, is detected using muscle testing and then magnets, using these same points to treat it.

Using magnets therapeutically like this retrains the immune system to properly address different pathogens. After the magnets are applied to the points corresponding to pathogens, over the next several months a protocol of nutritional support and a detox regimen is followed. At a follow-up visit after six months, the same procedure is done to check and treat any remaining infections. The technique is noninvasive and relies on your own immune system to perform the treatment as opposed to an external intervention using therapeutics. It is also gentle and only contraindicated for those who have pacemakers and for pregnant women (due to the release of toxins from pathogen die-off that can occur).

PEMF

Pulsed magnetic field therapy (PEMF) can be helpful for people with chronic Lyme Disease as it gives you the power to drive the remedies into the cells. It helps the functioning of your body as the muscles generate an electromagnetic charge and helps the macrophages and anti-inflammatory cells to do their job. PEMF reduces both inflammation and pain and improves circulation. It also increases the oxygen in the blood flow and helps to open cell membrane channels, allowing medications, supplements, and herbal remedies to be more effective. PEMF sessions are available through experienced practitioners, or given a larger budget, many devices such as the FDA-approved BEMER mat are available to the consumer.

GROUNDING

Grounding is the practice of literally putting one's bare feet on the earth whether it be sand, dirt, or grass. When walking barefoot on the earth, the body picks up free ions from the earth's surface which act as antioxidants in your body. Grounding might be the simplest and cheapest practice; however, the benefits, which range from decreased inflammation, decreased anxiety, to improved sleep, are profound. Twenty-one peer-reviewed published articles describe the benefits of grounding to lower inflammation specifically demonstrating that twenty minutes of grounding decreases cellular inflammation by 20 percent. Another eight-week study showed improved sleep and decreased stress levels when participants practiced grounding daily (Oschman 2015). The documentary *The Earthing Movie: The Remarkable Science of Grounding* gives an accessible and high-level overview of the science (Tickell and Tickell 2019). Unfortunately, most of the rubber-soled shoes that we wear insulate us from touching the earth and prevent the body from receiving free electrons. However, copper pegs can be placed in any pair of shoes to obtain a grounding effect. There are also several companies commercializing shoes and bed sheets that provide some benefit.

NEUROPLASTICITY

"Chronic illness is a bad habit of the brain."

—DR. DIETRICH KLINGHARDT

Your brain can get stuck in old patterns that can cause all kinds of physical and psychological symptoms. The more you focus on those symptoms, the more those patterns get solidified in your brain. Neuroplasticity is the ability of nerve synapses to regrow based on learned behavior. Branches that relay sensory information are pruned back to maintain efficiency. To regain or reinforce a certain function, you should expose yourself to the desired experience. Repeating the experience over time and on a recurring basis sends a signal that these neurons are necessary. Using the principles of neuroplasticity, your brain's ability to create new neural pathways, you can actually cause your brain to stop using those old pathways and use the new ones (Hopper 2014). Certain symptoms can be due to the negative reinforcement of old patterns. Additionally, there are systems, such as NeuroQuant, that can actually measure limbic system dysfunction which analyzes a brain MRI and determines stress based on the size of the amygdala—the part of our brain that processes emotions and memories associated with fear. So neuroplasticity can be used to correct old lingering symptoms, long after microbes are no longer being problematic.

Programs like Dynamic Neural Retraining System (DNRS) use this principle to help people with lingering and stubborn symptoms that haven't seen improvement with other therapies. The DNRS program runs for six months online and requires a commitment of one hour a day. Many physicians will recommend the program even if you cannot dedicate one hour a day; for example, fifteen minutes can have an impact. Apart from this time, you will need to become aware throughout your day of what kind of patterns you are encouraging in your mind. It requires you to implement what you learn in the course daily. Since DNRS, numerous other programs have been created.

For those who are unable to invest the time in a program like DNRS or other programs that involve a certain level of time commitment, there are alternatives, such as Cereset and Low Energy Neurofeedback System (LENS) therapy where the retraining or resetting is performed to you, as opposed to practicing on a recurring basis and engaging in an active training process. Cereset uses patented technology that listens to an individual's brain waves and plays it back to the person with sound. As the brain "hears" itself, it begins to relax and rebalance. This method is backed by peer-reviewed research and clinical trials; the actual treatment takes place over several days at one of the Cereset locations across the United States. Another modality is LENS which consists of a software program that is connected to an FDA-approved EEG device that measures brain waves and stimulates biochemical changes through radio waves applied through electrodes. The person doesn't feel or do anything other than sit still in a chair while a brief, tiny signal is applied to the brain. It is called *low energy* since the radio frequency waves are thousands of times weaker than what your brain is exposed to, for example, with a cellular phone close to your head. In a session, these radio waves are applied to certain areas of the head that correspond to different functions of the brain. Both Cereset and LENS appeal to people who cannot meet the time commitment of DNRS. The software and technology for both are available only at places equipped and guided by a certified practitioner. Both treatments are safe, and many people report relief of symptoms after multiple sessions, such as improved anxiety, mood, memory, sleep, and less PTSD. There are many other neural retraining techniques, such as Quantum Neuro Reset Therapy (QNRT) with the help of a chiropractor that works by resetting the brain from emotional shocks and trauma lodged in the nervous system. It uses applied kinesiology and a cold handheld laser to determine which parts of the brain are out of balance, and then a variety of tools are used to reset those nervous system pathways. For those looking for self-guided online options beyond DNRS, the Gupta program focuses on reengaging with joy and aims to retrain the amygdala. Another online application is BrainTap which can also be helpful to reset your limbic system.

Whatever your needs are, neuroplasticity or neural retraining is an emerging field, and now many options exist with varying degrees of efficacy for different individuals.

The field has gotten a lot of attention in recent years and more methods will likely emerge. Some people will reserve neural retraining until after treatment as the results may not be as long lasting or *sticky*, and other people prefer the body to prioritize energy for healing and supporting immune function. Depending on your needs, there is likely a neural retaining option that could work for you. If you haven't experienced relief of certain symptoms after multiple rounds of antimicrobial treatment, you might want to consider neuroplasticity.

TRAUMA HEALING

"No cure that fails to engage our spirits can make us well."
—VIKTOR FRANKL

There is a finite limit on healing your full being with only physical intervention. In fact, many people leave the emotional or mental part of healing last but later regret not prioritizing it earlier in their treatment. However, emotional trauma influences physical health in ways that are hard to appreciate. In fact, Dietrich Klinghardt, MD, PhD, who has been treating Lyme and chronic illness for more than thirty years, believes there is a correlation between how much toxicity and infection the individual harbors with how much trauma they carry. Trauma can be thought of as any experience that exceeds the person's ability to cope and that the individual is unable to process the emotions as part of the experience itself. Dr. Gabor Maté notes that "trauma is not what happens to us, it's what happens within us, as a result of what happened to us" (*When the Body Says No* 2003). Nearly all human beings have unresolved trauma, impacting our health in ways we don't even realize. In fact, a famous study by the CDC and Kaiser Permanente found that approximately 67 percent of adults have been exposed to trauma (Felitti et al. 1998). In Dr. Gabor Maté's book *When the Body Says No*, the mechanisms of how trauma can suppress immune function and affect cellular function are described at length. In another book, *The Body Keeps the Score*, the author Bessel van der Kolk describes how traumatic memories are different from other life events in that traumas are remembered as if they are being experienced again. The author learned this perspective by working with Vietnam War veterans, helping them reintegrate into society upon returning from war. He observed that trauma affects the normal functioning of the brain, allowing the emotional part of the brain to override the rational part of the brain—the prefrontal cortex—which creates stress or anxiety where the person is not able to live in the present (van der Kolk 2014). In summary, trauma impacts the immune system function and can hamper certain organs. Fortunately, there are tools to address trauma that are proven to work. First, let's take a look at the main types of trauma that could be problematic.

CHILDHOOD

The way a child experiences the world in the early years up until seven years old is quite different compared to adults. Indeed, it has been shown that adverse childhood events

(ACEs) can play a factor later in life and can set the stage for disease. At the time of writing, there are over 1,200 peer-reviewed studies on the relationship between childhood stress and adult illness. Research on this topic started in 1996 with the Kaiser Permanente-CDC Adverse Childhood Experiences Study, known as the ACE Study. In the words of Bessel van der Kolk, the ability to feel safe is "probably the most important aspect of mental health" (*The Body Keeps the Score* 2014). So when we grow up with family dynamics that make us feel unsafe, we can struggle to move past our personal and familial trauma.

GENERATIONAL

It has been shown that generational trauma can play a part in how an individual manages illness. Most research as it relates to trauma and epigenetics is conducted by observing trauma with mice and then observing how the next generation of mice respond to trauma. Then markers associated with mental illness and PTSD, such as the FKBP5 gene along with others that affect methylation and immune function, are tracked (Wilker 2014). As the book *It Didn't Start with You* by Mark Wolynn describes, in mouse models, it is observed that trauma can be traced back to six generations (2016).

Beyond animal models, researchers have observed the effects of events in history on individuals and their subsequent generations. For example, the 2018 research paper in the *Proceedings of the National Academy of Sciences* by three members of the Economics of Aging program at the National Bureau of Economics and Research in Cambridge, Massachusetts, revealed that the sons of imprisoned soldiers from the Civil War were far more likely to die of an untimely death than soldiers from that same era who were not imprisoned. Studies have also documented different dysregulated stress responses being passed down from survivors of the Holocaust and Dutch famine to grandchildren (Costa et al. 2018). Around the world, some cultures have recognized the importance of addressing trauma and have developed specific practices. For example, the late founder of Family Constellation Therapy found that in some traditions, there are ceremonies to prevent intergenerational trauma such as in the Zulu culture in southern Africa. After there is a murder in a Zulu community, the family of the deceased would make peace with the murderer. In other cultures, this might be known as breaking bread.

WHAT TO DO

Even being chronically ill is a traumatic experience in and of itself, going from doctor to doctor being told that it's all in your head and feeling like you are spinning your wheels not making progress with practitioners, not to mention the psycho-emotional symptoms that can torment you. Indeed, many with Lyme develop a sort of PTSD around their symptoms and have anxiety about relapses. So if you are human, you have likely experienced trauma, and your experience with Lyme may have added another traumatic layer. Fortunately, there is more and more research into the impact of trauma and also what to do about it. Talk therapy can be helpful but is limited in that it does not break out of the pattern of reliving the trauma to bring the person into present reality. Forms of therapy that attempt to address trauma may even be harmful as they may encourage the person to relive the experience. So for dealing with trauma, there are multiple options, such as Eye Movement Desensitization and Reprocessing (EMDR) and internal family systems

(IFS) with more emerging every day. EMDR, for example, is a form of trauma therapy that can have a significant impact on people to help process their healing experience. EMDR is effective and endorsed by the WHO, Department of Defense, and other well-recognized organizations. Various randomized controlled clinical studies have evaluated EMDR therapy; in one particular study, 80 percent of trauma victims no longer had PTSD after several ninety-minute sessions (Shapiro 2014; Wilson et al. 1995; Wilson et al. 1997; Rothbaum 1997).

There is also IFS developed by Richard C. Schwartz in the 1980s. IFS views the mind as made up of relatively discrete subpersonalities, each with its own unique viewpoint and qualities. A concept that makes IFS stand out from other approaches is that there are no bad or negative "parts." They are simply behaviors that form out of necessity almost as a protection mechanism. These behaviors then persist even after the person is out of the situation that provoked them or when they are no longer useful. Family constellation therapy is another promising therapy. Developed by the German therapist Bert Hellinger, a family constellation attempts to reveal a dynamic that spans multiple generations in a family and to resolve the effects of that dynamic. As the science of epigenetics has now proven, these events can exert a powerful force affecting future generations. Another emerging field for trauma therapy is psychedelics. At the time of writing, some of the most respected scientists and researchers in institutions such as Johns Hopkins, UCLA, and NYU are making progress with psychedelic-assisted therapy for treating a variety of mental health disorders (Gukasyan et al. 2022; Martinez 2022). With legalization currently in a number of states in the United States and the work of the Multidisciplinary Association for Psychedelic Studies (MAPS), a nonprofit organization working to raise awareness and understanding of psychedelic substances, demonstrating efficacy in clinical trials, this new modality is expected to be more widely available in the coming years as the science and regulation move forward. Sometimes the trauma is unclear, and you may not realize that certain life events have affected you in profound ways. Applied Psycho-Neurobiology (APN) developed by Dr. Dietrich Klinghardt in the 1980s is a combination of techniques used to address multiple levels of healing including the nonphysical, the mental body, and the intuitive body in this framework. Through APN, the trauma event can be identified along with which organs are impacted and the accompanying emotions associated with the event. By understanding the frequencies and the organs involved, the effect can be reset with the help of an experienced practitioner. This therapy is especially useful for those who do not identify or remember the trauma.

7

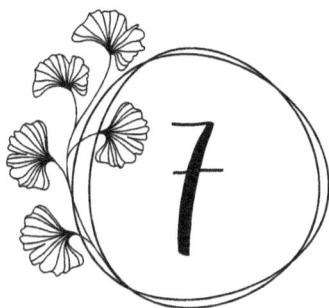

DETOX AND DRAINAGE

"Give me six hours to chop down a tree and I will spend the first four sharpening the axe."

—ABRAHAM LINCOLN

During treatment of Lyme, your body is producing a lot of neurotoxins or endotoxins from bacteria die-off. A common mistake is focusing so much on the killing and not enough on getting what's being killed out. Industrialized toxins, Lyme Disease toxins from the microbes themselves, buildup of synthetic drugs or supplements, and stress from chronic illness mean that people with Lyme Disease have a higher concentration of accumulated toxins in their body than most people. So already, your detox pathways are likely working overtime and the importance of detox cannot be understated. A person's ability to clear toxins is also due to emotional stress, genetics, lifestyle choices, level of infection, and continued exposure to toxins. Additionally, Lyme inhibits many enzymes needed by the body for detox.

So how much detox is too much? The simple answer is that you will know it as you'll feel it. When you release more toxins than your body can handle, you might be detoxing too much. The recommendation would be to back off. The extent to which you can tolerate treatment corresponds to your ability to eliminate and circulate excess toxins.

TERRAIN FOCUS

Throughout history, there has been debate about the source of chronic disease. Is the pathogen to blame or the environment that allows the pathogen to thrive? A key differentiating factor between naturopathic and conventional medicine is the focus on the body's terrain—the environment in your body that hosts the pathogen. Dating back to the 1800s, the germ theory promoted by Louis Pasteur has had a profound effect on the course of modern medicine. However, the other school of thought that was shared by Pasteur's colleague, Claude Bernard, agrees with Hippocrates, that our body's "terrain" is primarily responsible for chronic disease. The terrain, or biological terrain as many people refer to it, is thought of as the overall environment, like the soil that feeds and nourishes the cells in the body. The debate between these two schools of thought continues today. Although it is worth noting that after all the back-and-forth between these two groups, Pasteur acknowledged the importance of the terrain on his deathbed, admitting, "Claude Bernard was right...The microbe is nothing; the terrain is everything." Two hundred years later, modern medicine continues to ignore this wisdom and focuses on killing microorganisms when what many people need most is a more functional terrain to rebalance the body. The following sections focus on this topic and on opening up the detox pathways, the channels that your body uses to eliminate toxins, and on supporting the function of the relevant organs in the process.

LIVER SUPPORT

From the Anglo-Saxon word for liver, *lifer*, it seems logical that the etymology of the word *liver* is related to "life." The German word for liver is *die Leber*, and the verb *leben* is "to live." The liver is an impressive workhorse and central to clearing the body of pathogens and toxins. The liver holds half the body's blood supply at any given time and is the second largest organ and responsible for hundreds of functions in the body, including cleaning the blood, generating lymph, producing hormones, generating bile, absorbing nutrients, and breaking down toxins, among many other functions. For Lyme detox, the liver plays a central role as it tags toxins meant to leave the body and sends them to the digestive tract and kidneys for removal. Although liver cells regenerate every three months, to think that its capabilities regenerate to its original function is an incorrect assumption. When someone is dealing with chronic illness and an overburdened liver, bile production goes from its normal 800 ml to 1,000 ml a day to a cup or less. This decreased capacity affects a person's detox ability to excrete fat-soluble vitamins. So supporting your liver on a continual basis is crucial, potentially exploring liver flushes or cleanses as well.

LIVER FLUSH

There are many different versions of a liver flush, but essentially it consists of following a nourishing vegetarian diet with minimal fats, juices, and soups to prepare the body to eliminate and the liver to work, using liver-supportive herbs and finally using oil, usually olive, to flush out waste matter. An apple cider tonic with lemon and cayenne pepper is also used to prepare and soften waste material. Herbs that might be involved are chanca piedra and gold coin grass that help break up "stones" or hardened matter that may clog bile ducts. *The Amazing Liver and Gallbladder Flush* by Andreas Moritz goes into detail about how to perform a liver flush (1998). It is worth mentioning that just because this process is a natural intervention that doesn't use pharmaceutical drugs, it does not mean a liver flush is harmless. There are actually several important risks in doing a liver flush. It is very important to follow the guidance of an experienced practitioner who has been trained and qualified to lead people through a liver flush and be aware that it can be contraindicated for certain people, especially when dealing with gallstones, in a treatment pro-tocol or with a weakened constitution. Apart from the liver flush itself, you can support your liver on an ongoing basis by eating liver-supportive foods, such as beets, dandelion greens, artichoke, and onions (Cabot 1997). To help with digestion, it is recommended to start eating with an acid such as apple cider vinegar and incorporating bitters. Sometimes when you're in a cleanse and need to be mindful of your liver, avoiding foods that are hard to digest such as red meat is advised.

CASTOR-OIL PACK

When castor oil is applied topically over the abdomen, it is absorbed through the skin into the tissues. With the use of heat, it helps drive the oil even deeper so it's able to increase lymphocyte production and increase the circulation of the lymphatic system. Using it over the liver also stimulates the liver to dump bile. Castor-oil packs are a practice that you can incorporate on a regular basis with little to no downside. The process is very gentle, so if you feel sensitive to more intense detox practices, you might consider applying a castor-oil pack for only twenty minutes. It is important that high-quality organic castor oil is used along with an organic cloth.

BOWEL MOTILITY

Toxins are released through exhalation, sweat, urine, and bowel movements. There are two types of toxins: water soluble and fat soluble. The kidneys handle the water-soluble toxins, while the liver primarily handles the fat-soluble ones. A golden rule throughout treatment is that you should be having at least one daily bowel movement, and if for some reason this is not the case, you should take measures to make it happen.

Here are some reasons why you might be struggling with bowel motility and corresponding solutions.

ROOT CAUSE	SUGGESTIONS
Liver congestion (from the reduction or stoppage of bile flow or otherwise known as cholestasis)	Bile acids serve as a laxative to move stagnant bile. Bitters, TUDCA, and butyrate can also be helpful.
Lack of hydration	Stools are 75 percent water, so you should drink your weight in ounces divided by two. Also, incorporate minerals and trace elements such as Quinton electrolytes.
Food sensitivities	Avoid food sensitivities and implement a plan to reduce leaky gut.
Disrupted microbiome	Use a potent probiotic or a spore-based probiotic like MegaSpore and consume enough fiber. Although we don't know the exact quantity of fiber that humans ate thousands of years ago, at least 30 mg of a mix of insoluble and soluble fiber is a good benchmark.
Parasites	It is recommended to work with a practitioner on a parasite cleanse.
Reduced vagal tone	This can happen with Lyme and coinfections and also in the case of trauma.
Lack of exercise or inactivity	Exercise speeds up the time it takes for food to pass through the large intestine. Walking even ten to fifteen minutes several times a day is helpful. Aerobic exercise like running, swimming, or dancing speeds up your breathing and heart rate which helps to stimulate the natural contractions of the intestine muscles.

There are other causes and underlying illnesses not covered here, such as hemorrhoids or colon cancer.

If you have tried the above suggestions and haven't had any luck, there are a few supplements worth mentioning that can help as temporary support, such as Bowel Mover by CellCore or magnesium oxide supplements, or even vitamin C, coffee, cacao, or prunes. Look for changes in lifestyle or supplements that could be the cause, such as not exercising or moving enough or overusing binders. Colonics and coffee enemas can also change your elimination patterns and disrupt normal intestinal and colon flora.

BINDERS

Additionally, you can consider binders, such as activated charcoal, bentonite clay, zeolite powder, and citrus pectin specifically to help with elimination of endotoxins and prevent their recirculation. When you are using binders regardless of which binders are used, toxins will be picked up and a portion of them will be dropped. Unfortunately, there's no way to get around this. Even though some binders are better than others in this sense, simply be aware that you might feel toxins moving around when taking binders. Each binder has specific usages: zeolite for petrochemicals, and humic and fulvic acid for ammonia released by parasites and other bacterial by-products, for example. Combination binders can be helpful, such as GI Detox by Biocidin and Ultra Binder by Quicksilver Scientific. Work with a practitioner to incorporate these and make sure to take binders at least two hours away from other medication. Charcoal should be used on a temporary basis only because it binds up fatty acids and other precious nutrients, whereas chlorella tends to not bind up as many nutrients and is better for more long-term use. When choosing binders, sourcing is extremely important as algae, clays, and charcoal can be contaminated with toxins themselves, so cheapening out can actually be worse. Although binders can provide relief of symptoms, be mindful that they do not affect your cadence of elimination. Overuse can lead to constipation, which one should avoid at all cost during treatment.

VAGUS NERVE SUPPORT

People can go a long time attributing symptoms to other infections when in reality, what is causing many of their symptoms may be a toxic or malfunctioning vagus nerve. The vagus nerve may be malfunctioning due to toxicity or infection, which may compromise many functions including digestion, detox, recovery, pain regulation, and respiration. The word *vagus* means wandering in Latin, appropriate for this nerve which is the longest cranial nerve in the body and runs all the way from the brain stem to part of the colon. It modulates most of the activity of the autonomic nervous system. Over time, it can be affected by Lyme and coinfections along with dental infections. The healthier this nerve is, the higher the vagal tone and the quicker your body is able to relax.

Potential symptoms of vagus nerve damage or distinction include:

- Difficulty speaking or loss of voice
- Hoarse or wheezy voice
- Trouble drinking liquids
- Loss of the gag reflex
- Pain in the ear
- Unusual heart rate
- Abnormal blood pressure
- Decreased production of stomach acid
- Nausea or vomiting
- Abdominal bloating or pain

There are various measures that can correct and help support proper vagal tone:

- Craniosacral therapy
- Vagus nerves exercises as described in Stanley Rosenberg's book *Accessing the Healing Power of the Vagus* (2017)
- Cold exposure
- Deep and slow breathing
- Singing, humming, chanting, and gargling
- Probiotics or a gut-repair protocol
- Meditation
- Omega-3 fatty acids
- Exercise
- Massage
- Deep belly breathing
- Sleeping on right side

In addition to these measures, there are vagus nerve stimulation devices which are electrical devices that may stimulate the nerve, using ear clips attached to the neck area below the ear lobes at the start of the vagus nerve. A program called BrainTap claims to support vagal tone along with emotional freedom technique (EFT).

DETOX MODALITIES

Many Lyme practitioners recommend "detox as if it is your job" by rotating in and out different detox modalities daily. The following options are listed in order of both effectiveness and intensity.

SAUNA

Unfortunately, Lyme bacteria don't die until the heat reaches around 106°F while some of the coinfections such as *Bartonella* are more heat sensitive. In fact, there is a form of therapy that uses heat, along with antibiotics, to kill microbes called hyperthermia where the body is heated to around 107°F. This process is done very slowly, under close monitoring and supervision, as it carries many risks. However, the purpose of using a sauna is primarily for detox. Heat can make the bacteria start to move and in doing so make them more accessible to antibiotic treatment or to the immune system. It is also advisable to take your antimicrobials within one hour after your sauna. The sauna pushes the spirochetes into the bloodstream and out of the deep tissues, where they can then be more easily killed by your antimicrobial remedies. It is also advisable to use binders as many toxins will be mobilized. The surface area of the gut is about the size of a tennis court when spread out, compared to the surface area of the skin which is only a few square meters. When sweating in a sauna, the gut is going through a similar process of excreting toxins. So if you don't use a binder, these toxins get reabsorbed. To avoid this reabsorption, you can use a binder, for example chlorella or zeolite, an hour before so that the gut is lined with the binder. Apart from the support with your Lyme detox protocol, saunas have many benefits including easing muscle pain, lessening inflammation, improving mental clarity, easing anxiety and depression, and other cardiovascular benefits.

Start low and slow with saunas. Then you can work up to around three per week, ten to fifteen minutes at first, then up to twenty to thirty minutes. Use a towel intermittently to wipe your sweat and quickly shower when you finish to rinse the sweat so the toxins are not reabsorbed through the skin. It is also recommended to use a cold shower afterward to close pores so the toxins are not reabsorbed. Make sure to replenish electrolytes. Deep sea minerals and Quinton electrolytes can be great options. If you don't have access to a sauna, there are many infrared saunas that you can buy. An important factor when looking for saunas is to watch for risk of non-native EMF. Portable or at-home saunas are a good option and are not as expensive as you would expect. Therasage and Sunlighten are reputable brands with a high level of quality. They both offer low-EMF/VOC models. These portable smaller saunas can be bought for around $1,500.

MOVING LYMPH

Stagnation is the best friend of Lyme, so it is important that you keep moving. Even though the lymphatic system plays such an important role in our bodies with much more fluid than the cardiovascular system, it is one of the most overlooked systems of the body. It removes toxins and waste from the body, so when the lymph gets congested, toxins build up within the body and impede cell function. Some people use lymphatic massage, a small trampoline, walking at least half an hour per day, and dry skin brushing which helps detoxify your skin by increasing blood circulation and promoting lymph flow. Also, homeopathy remedies such as Itires provide coverage for the kidneys, liver, and lymphatic system.

COFFEE ENEMA

A common misconception is thinking that coffee enemas support the colon when in reality, their major effect is on the liver. When you fill an enema up with coffee and start to let it flow, the hemorrhoid veins absorb the caffeine. From there, it goes up to the portal vein which carries it up to the liver and gallbladder. Once the liver receives the caffeine and palmitic acids, it immediately reacts because the caffeine is an irritant to the liver. This action makes the liver open its bile ducts and start dumping bile out quickly. Since toxins are stored in the liver, this process of draining the bile from the liver dumps all of it out into the stomach so it can be shuttled out of the body. A lot of people resist trying coffee enemas, but the effect of bile movement and liver support to help mobilize toxins is immediately impactful and overwhelmingly beneficial. Coffee enemas also produce a burst of glutathione.

Although coffee is overly beneficial, according to a recent study for example, coffee contains twenty-one metabolites that are liver protective (Loftfield et al. 2020). Coffee can be dehydrating if you're not used to it. If you're doing coffee enemas frequently, make sure you are taking trace minerals and adequately hydrating. A good practice is doing a pre and post enema with water or aloe vera to prevent dehydration and ensure a more complete elimination. Be sure to buy organic coffee, specifically for enema use. Coffee enemas can be time consuming, so there are alternatives, such as coffee bean suppositories which can have a similar positive impact while minimizing the time commitment and also minimizing the impact on disrupting colon floral, which one should be mindful of with frequent coffee enema use.

COLON HYDROTHERAPY

The average person has between 5 and 10 kg of impacted fecal matter in their colon. Although a coffee enema may reach the descending part of the colon, a colon hydrotherapy session or a colonic reaches the entire colon. Colon hydrotherapy is a method of removing waste from the large intestine without the use of drugs or chemicals. A session involves diluting and removing toxins from the colon resulting in improved digestion and overall health. It may help with chronic constipation, diarrhea, bloating, gas, and sluggish metabolism/digestive problems.

IONIC FOOTBATH

The ionic footbath is a physical bath that you soak your feet in while a low-voltage electric current charges the atoms in the water molecules which are then meant to attract and neutralize negatively charged toxins. So a direct current goes through one end of an array of the footbath, through the water, and back through the other end of the array. This toxin removal process is believed to positively charge the hydrogen present in the water. This positive charge then attracts the negatively charged toxins present in your body. During the footbath, the water begins to change color naturally because of the chemical reaction between the electricity and the salt water, not because of toxins, which is a common misconception. The toxins are not dumped into the tub of water, so it's not important what is in the water or what color the water is. After the footbath itself, over the next several days, the body will be excreting toxins. The ionic footbath is a hotly debated topic as there are few independent large studies on its effectiveness. Some studies discredit the footbath citing that there is no significant difference of toxins in the water. On the other hand, a study in 2008 by the Center for Research Strategies found that in the thirty-one participants who underwent ionic detox two times per week for twelve weeks, the average blood level of aluminum decreased by 46 percent, and the average blood level of arsenic decreased by 24 percent after the twelve weeks (Wass and Gallagher 2008). In many other cases, studies have been done to sample the urine before and after the footbath and the urine showed orders of magnitude in excretion of toxins for days after the footbath. The reader is invited to check out the literature available, review the contraindications, which include pacemakers, certain heart problems, and epilepsy, for instance, and also speak to a doctor to decide whether footbaths are right for your situation.

MASSAGE

Massage can increase blood flow to muscle tissues and make antibiotics access hard-to-reach areas. If you are new to massage, start with a shorter, light session like less than thirty minutes, then slowly work up to a longer, more intensive session which may produce herx reactions. Even if you can't get to a session, you can practice self-massage, especially around the thyroid (to support hypothyroid tendencies, overall thyroid health, release toxins from the teeth, help venous drainage, etc.), as well as breast and liver for general drainage.

CRANIOSACRAL THERAPY

Few systems in the body have more impact on the central nervous system than the craniosacral system, which consists of the soft tissue and fluid that protect, feed, and detox our brain and spinal cord. Craniosacral therapy releases restrictions caused over time from toxins, infections, injury, and other stressors and allows the entire body to relax, unwind, and self-correct. This gentle type of manual therapy can create dramatic improvements and releases restrictions deep in the body to relieve dysfunction and pain.

EPSOM SALT BATH

Epsom salt baths are a gentle way to detox, with two or three cups of Epsom salt in a warm bath. Be mindful of the temperature as a very hot bath can provoke die-off since hot temperatures can make the microbes move out of tissues. Add baking soda (a clean product without any aluminum) to your bath to help the magnesium absorb better. Epsom salt baths can also help with oxalates. If you are bathing daily or frequently, it is recommended that you use a shower filter so you avoid absorbing toxins from the municipal water through your skin.

BREATHING

Many people have developed a habit of breathing in the upper part of the lungs instead of deeply from the diaphragm due to stress and out of habit. Shallower breathing restricts oxygen flow and the release of toxins. Fortunately, this habit can be corrected with yoga, breathing exercises, and meditation. The more deeply we breathe, the more waste we release and the more we reduce the negative physiological effects of stress on our bodies. The body is more acidic in the morning, so alkalinizing has a huge benefit in the morning and also helps the mitochondria. There is more and more science that indicates disease is encouraged with an acidic body. So activities that can help alkalize your body will help put it in a state of higher function. The Wim Hof breathing or pranayama, for example, can alkalize your body effectively.

This list is only a sample of the many detox modalities available. As the Lyme microbes become less problematic and you advance in your treatment, the need to detox will decrease. Although detox is a lifelong commitment, now you are armed with this knowledge for whenever the need arises to move toxins through your body effectively or to better support your body's own detox abilities.

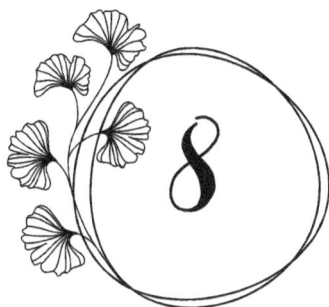

RECOVERY

"The wound is the place where the light enters you."

—RUMI

REPAIR AND REGENERATION

After various microbes are eliminated, symptoms may still persist that are not due to microbe activity but from remaining damage and dysfunction. Dead bacteria particles will need to be removed and eliminated, so continuing detox practices after your treatment protocol is advisable. Also, enough toxins, which your own body will produce from killing pathogens along with external toxins, in particular, mold, can cause immune dysregulation. So for this additional reason, even after your immune system has addressed pathogens, you should still continue good detox practices. As reviewed in the neuroplasticity section, dysregulation can cause your nervous system to be stuck in old patterns, and it is recommended to readers that they review neural retraining options in this case. Many practitioners observe that the time it takes your body to repair damage will correlate roughly to how long you have been sick. This rule of thumb is a generalization and certainly doesn't apply to everyone but reflects the time that it might take to heal. Almost every cell in your body can be completely regenerated in seven to ten years (with exception of the brain cells behind your eyes which your body keeps forever). So your body will regenerate in time with some organs taking longer to heal; the brain, for example, can take up to a year to heal.

Unfortunately, killing the troublesome microbes does not immediately equate to restoring health. By combining some of the therapies and practices reviewed in this book, you will support your body to fully recover and become more resilient to future challenges. Autophagy, the state induced by fasting, can also help "clean up" and repair damage done by infections or pathogens. Fasting or fasting-mimicking diets can be helpful, even trying a more ketogenic diet. There are many helpful remedies that can be useful such as phospholipids for cell wall repair and a multivitamin to cover any remaining nutritional deficiencies. Many people will also be low in secretory Ig, so supplementing with colostrum can replenish stores that have been depleted chronically. Collagen is a good idea as it will support healing joints and connective tissue that may have been affected.

Many people who have gone through this process develop an immense gratitude and humbleness. However, depending on one's experience with the illness and treatment, trauma around the illness itself and neuroplasticity can be real factors to recovery. Many people struggle with recognizing and addressing the trauma of feeling unsafe or overwhelmed with fear when experiencing symptoms, not to mention the frustration and abandonment from navigating the conventional medical system.

REINFECTION

It just takes one bite to be reinfected with Lyme and coinfections. The probability of reinfection is affected in large part by many lifestyle factors, such as where one lives, the frequency that one is outdoors, and one's precautions and awareness with regard to being in nature. A reinfection might feel like a resurgence of old symptoms. The symptoms might feel the same as before, or they might be slightly different depending on the species of the coinfection. It might come on subtlety or abruptly. A common belief held among Lyme practitioners and those who have been through the illness is that the majority of the population has been exposed to vector-borne infections like Lyme at some point. However, they are unaffected or asymptomatic. What makes the difference as to whether one suffers symptoms is the constitution and overall body burden as described in previous sections. Depending on what your exposure to insect bites is, you may rethink protective measures including the ones mentioned earlier in this book and more intentionally incorporate them into daily life.

MAINTENANCE VERSUS REMISSION

There is much discussion as to what defines remission as there is no test that is universally used by practitioners to determine whether someone is done with treatment or whether someone is in remission, as explained in the testing section. Some practitioners don't use the word *remission*, whereas others consider that sufficient time without having active symptoms as remission. Generally, the following points are taken into account when determining whether someone is in remission or not:

- **Symptom relief.** There may be leftover symptoms due to repair that's needed. However, active symptoms are not presenting for several months. Practitioners vary in opinions about the time span to be symptom-free.
- **High natural killer (NK) cell count.** A sufficiently high NK or CD57 count is at least 150 or higher.
- **Testing.** In addition to the labs mentioned in the testing chapter, many people also find muscle testing with an experienced practitioner useful to determine if microbial stressors are still present.
- **Antibodies.** Presence of antibodies shows that your body mounted a response.

If the body is still dealing with an active infection or unable to keep the microbes in check, any procedure or event where your body may experience significant stress, physical or mental, could present an opportunity for reactivation. The studies have not been done in the scientific community to indicate what factors trigger a reactivation of symptoms. However, from the experience of many people dealing with Lyme, together with experienced practitioners, mold exposure, surgeries possibly exposing areas harboring microbes, parasitic infections can trigger a reactivation, and even major emotional stressors can trigger a reactivation.

CONCLUSION

After you finish reading this book, your head might be exploding with new information or you might feel overwhelmed. You also might be wondering, where do I begin? Or you might be frustrated that there is not one clear path to recovery or pill that is guaranteed to work for everyone. Or you might also be intimidated by concepts that you don't necessarily understand or that have been otherwise debunked by the medical community at large.

I suggest you start by reminding yourself that you *can* get well and that you actively nurture a sense of hope wherever you are in your journey. Throughout this book, we've gone through many levers that you can use from sleep, diet, movement, stress, and environment to your emotions that will profoundly impact your healing outcomes. Only you have the control to make changes in these areas. Every day, you make hundreds of decisions about the food you consume and the environment you surround yourself with. So you should feel empowered as you are in the driver's seat. You also now have more insight into how complex treating Lyme and coinfections can be and how these pathogens affect the body. You are aware of the broader context and history of the disease and understand that the treatment and diagnostic tools are limited along with minimal public and private research. You are also aware that multiple treatment modalities or supportive therapies exist, in addition to pharmaceutical and herbal antibiotics, each with varying levels of efficacy and scientific rigor. Moreover, you recognize that these options are highly individualized and that what works for one person may not work for you, and so you appreciate the importance of trial and error. You also understand the importance of detox and that there are multiple modalities to choose from to support your body in eliminating toxins. *Lyme warriors* is the term used to refer to people dealing with Lyme, and the term reflects the tenacity required to get well. Healing is possible, but it is in your hands and your hands only.

The body is always trying to move toward health and has incredible capabilities to repair itself. The onion analogy is often used to describe this process, that layers need to be peeled off one by one, with certain pathogens or toxins only revealing themselves when your body is ready. Many people with Lyme have lived a lot of life, traveled to multiple places, had multiple jobs, or have a colorful family history or ancestry. They've taken multiple insults and their healing unravels in multiple layers. Like the proverbial onion analogy, when one layer is removed, another one shows itself.

Healing is not linear; it's a dynamic process.

WHAT WE *THINK* HEALING LOOKS LIKE

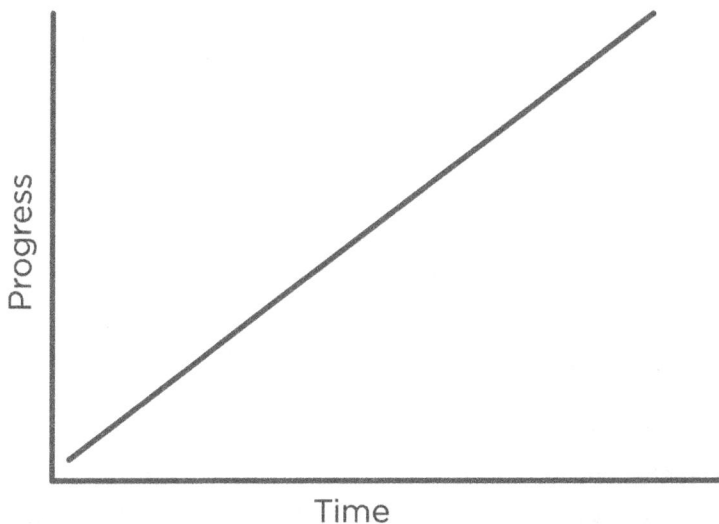

Progress / Time

WHAT HEALING *REALLY* LOOKS LIKE

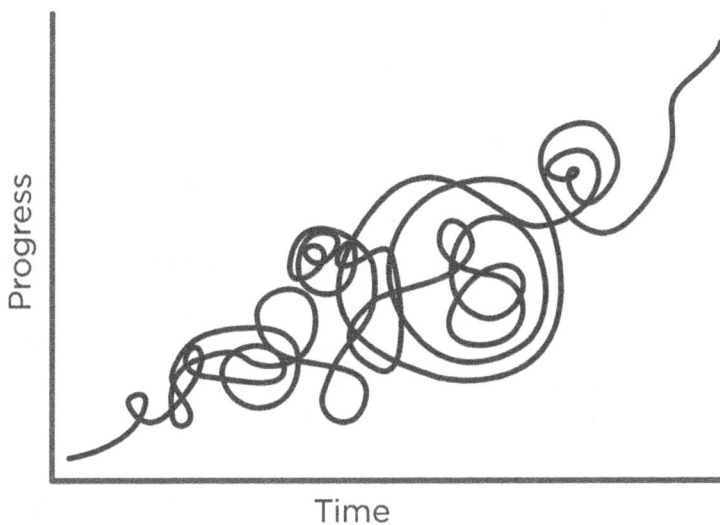

Progress / Time

There is also no timeline for healing from Lyme Disease. People heal at different speeds, so making a comparison between other people may be counterproductive. What makes someone turn the corner in terms of accelerating the healing progress may have little to no effect on you.

Whatever you did up until now got you to the point where you are at. Doing the same things will not produce different results. If you want change, it takes a level of commitment. So after going through your own healing journey, maybe you will see things through a new lens, which means in a lot of ways making decisions such as what to eat or more longer-term decisions such as where to live now have an additional layer of consideration. For example, it might take you longer to find a house, since you'd like to be away from major highways or power stations or only accept certain ERMI scores for mold levels. You might have made changes in your career as you realized that your previous job did not fulfill you and listening to your heart has an impact on your well-being. Also, you might continue detox practices and clean living beyond the Lyme treatment as you might have a new appreciation of how toxins affect a functional immune system. Based on the journey you have traveled, your commitment to living life on your own terms might have changed. Once you enter the rabbit hole of health and wellness, you start to realize that vibrancy and well-being does not necessarily have to go in a downward spiral as you age and that you can increasingly live a vibrant life full of joy and love. The tools you've learned throughout your healing journey will undoubtedly serve you in other areas of life. They will make you more resilient in the future to face stressors as they arrive, which includes healthy aging. In other words, these tools can help you increase your "health span" or the years of your life with good quality of life and wellness.

Losing your agency is among the worst experiences there is and chronic illness can be extremely overwhelming, especially when you cannot see the end of the tunnel and there is no one-and-done cure. Sometimes all you can think of is about how unfair life is. Giving up the activity or sport that you love, forgetting familiar names, observing your body age prematurely—these are things that can affect your quality of life in profound ways.

Keep trusting in the process and hang in there. It is possible to heal completely from Lyme and coinfections, and there is a beautiful life on the other side of this illness. With the confusion and lack of awareness around Lyme Disease within our communities, one may develop a tough skin and learn to trust one's instincts or intuition. Even loved ones may doubt and attribute symptoms to anxiety or mental health. Throughout the treatment process, one learns about the body and develops a heightened self-awareness. This wisdom and inner strength serves for the rest of one's life. Oftentimes, illness is an indication that a directional change needs to be made. You may have made many changes already or are in the process of profound change. Take a moment to recognize how far you have come and honor your efforts and courage.

On the other side of this healing journey, how you move, nourish yourself, play, fulfill your purpose, and who you spend your time with may change. This process can be a catalyst for personal growth, and it can change your perspective on life and your level of awareness about how your body is affected by the world. Illness is like a cocoon and the transformation is hard, but it's a beautiful thing that once set in motion cannot be reversed. Like a butterfly in a cocoon, one must face the struggle and only when ready, one may be free.

ACKNOWLEDGMENTS

Thank you to all the tireless doctors who work in the service of Lyme patients with such empathy and intellectual rigor.

I'm extremely grateful for having worked with a few of them, to name a few, Dr. April Blake for getting to the bottom of my health mystery after conventional medicine failed me and helping to guide me through much uncertainty. Dr. Klassen for being my local quarterback Lyme-literate doctor (LLMD), keeping me afloat through the rough patches of detox and Herx reactions with acupuncture sessions. Dr. Grieder who stuck with me through various treatment iterations, transitioning me to herbal and more holistic protocols. Dr. Deb and the team at Sophia Health Institute for all that they do.

And thanks to Dr. Tony Smith from LymeStop, who has been described by his many LymeStop patients as an earth angel, for restoring my hope and turning the corner for me. Thank you,

Dr. Tony, for developing such an elegant and beautiful therapy that is saving so many lives, including my own.

Thank you to the many doctors who also made me realize that I, and I alone, am responsible for my own well-being and health and that if I wanted to get well, I had to take matters into my own hands.

Thanks to my dear friends who showed up when I needed them and to my business partners and collaborators for their patience and understanding.

Thanks to my mom and my sister for trusting me when things got hairy and for all their patience and unconditional love.

Finally, infinite thanks to my dear love and partner in crime, Andrew, who had a front-row seat to my journey. I love you and I'm forever grateful for your unwavering support.

To all the wonderful humans and healers who helped me on my journey, I am immensely grateful, and I don't know how I would have navigated all of this without you.

REFERENCES

Bailey, Frazer, director. 2019. *Root Cause*. Netflix.

Beecher, Henry K. 1995. "The Powerful Placebo." *Journal of the American Medical Association* 157, no. 17. https://doi.org/10.1001/jama.1955.02960340022006.

Benson, Herbert, and Miriam Z. Kippler. 1976. *The Relaxation Response*. New York: William Morrow.

Bransfield, Robert C. 2018. "Neuropsychiatric Lyme Borreliosis: An Overview with a Focus on a Specialty Psychiatrist's Clinical Practice." *Healthcare* 6, no. 3 (September): 104. https://doi.org/10.3390/healthcare6030104.

Buhner, Stephen Harrod. 2012. *The Transformational Power of Fasting: The Way to Spiritual, Physical, and Emotional Rejuvenation*. Rochester, VT: Healing Arts Press.

———. 2015. *Healing Lyme: Natural Healing of Lyme Borreliosis and the Coinfections Chlamydia and Spotted Fever Rickettsioses*. Silver City, NM: Raven Press.

Cabello, Felipe C., Henry P. Godfrey, Julia V. Bugrysheva, and Stuart A. Newman. 2017. "Sleeper Cells: The Stringent Response and Persistence in the *Borreliella (Borrelia) burgdorferi* Enzootic Cycle." *Environmental Microbiology* 19, no. 10 (August): 3846–3862. https://doi.org/10.1111/1462-2920.13897.

Cabot, Sandra. 1997. *The Liver Cleansing Diet: Love Your Liver and Live Longer*. Scottsdale, AZ: S. C. B. International.

Cameron, Daniel J., Lorraine B. Johnson, and Elizabeth L. Maloney. 2014. "Evidence Assessments and Guideline Recommendations in Lyme Disease: The Clinical Management of Known Tick Bites, Erythema Migrans Rashes and Persistent Disease." *Expert Review of Anti-infective Therapy* 12, no. 9 (September): 1103–1130. https://doi.org/10.1586/14787210.2014.940900.

Carney, Scott. 2017. *What Doesn't Kill Us: How Freezing Water, Extreme Altitude, and Environmental Conditioning Will Renew Our Lost Evolutionary Strength*. New York: Rodale Books.

Centers for Disease Control and Prevention. 2021. "Lyme Disease Maps: Historical Data." Last reviewed April 30, 2021. https://www.cdc.gov/Lyme/stats/maps.html.

———. 2022. "Data and Surveillance." Last reviewed August 29, 2022. https://www.cdc.gov/lyme/datasurveillance/index.html?CDC_AA_refVal=https%3A%2F%2Fwww.cdc.gov%2Flyme%2Fstats%2Findex.html.

———. 2022. "Lyme Disease." Last reviewed January 19, 2022. https://www.cdc.gov/lyme/index.html.

Chesney, Alexis. 2020. *Preventing Lyme & Other Tick-Borne Diseases: Control Ticks in the Home Landscape; Prevent Infection Using Herbal Protocols; Treat Tick Bites with Natural Remedies*. North Adams, MA: Storey Publishing.

Choukér, Alexander, and Alexander C. Stahn. 2020. "COVID-19—The Largest Isolation Study in History: The Value of Shared Learnings from Spaceflight Analogs." *npj Microgravity* 6, no. 32. https://doi.org/10.1038/s41526-020-00122-8.

Consumer Reports. 2022. "Insect Repellents." Accessed October 10, 2022. https://www.consumerreports.org/products/insect-repellent-37160/insect-repellent-34772/view2/.

Costa, Dora L., Noelle Yetter, and Heather DeSomer. 2018. "Intergenerational Transmission of Paternal Trauma among US Civil War Ex-POWs." *PNAS* 115, no. 44 (October): 11215–11220. https://doi.org/10.1073/pnas.1803630115.

Crista, Jill. 2018. *Break the Mold: 5 Tools to Conquer Mold and Take Back Your Health*. Wellness Ink Publishing.

Dadd, Debra Lynn. 1990. *Nontoxic, Natural and Earthwise: How to Protect Yourself and Your Family from Harmful Products and Live in Harmony with the Earth*. Los Angeles: J. P. Tarcher.

DeBaun, Daniel T., and Ryan P. DeBaun. 2017. *Radiation Nation: The Fallout of Modern Technology*. Icaro Publishing.

Debelian, Gilberto Jirair, Ingar Olsen, and Leif Tronstad. 1998. "Anaerobic Bacteremia and Fungemia in Patients Undergoing Endodontic Therapy: An Overview." *Annals of Periodontology* 3, no. 1 (July): 281–287. https://doi.org/10.1902/annals.1998.3.1.281.

Emoto, Masaru. 2011. *The Hidden Messages in Water*. New York: Atria Books.

"Environment." 2022. Worldometer. Accessed December 6, 2022. https://www.worldometers.info/.

Fallon, Sally. 1999. *Nourishing Traditions: The Cookbook That Challenges Politically Correct Nutrition and the Diet Dictocrats*. Washington, DC: NewTrends Publishing.

Felitti, Vincent J., Robert F. Anda, Dale Nordenberg, David F. Williamson, Alison M. Spitz, Valerie Edwards, Mary P. Koss, and James S. Marks. 1998. "Relationship of Childhood Abuse and Household Dysfunction to Many of the Leading Causes of Death in Adults: The Adverse Childhood Experiences (ACE) Study." *American Journal of Preventive Medicine* 14, no. 4 (May): 245–258. https://doi.org/10.1016/S0749-3797(98)00017-8.

Feng, Jie, Jacob Leone, Sunjya Schweig, and Ying Zhang. 2020. "Evaluation of Natural and Botanical Medicines for Activity against Growing and Non-Growing Forms of *B. burgdorferi*." *Frontiers in Medicine* 7, no. 6 (February). https://doi.org/10.3389/fmed.2020.00006.

Forsgren, Scott. 2009. "Kryptopyrroluria (AKA Hemopyrrollactamuria): A Major Piece of the Puzzle in Overcoming Chronic Lyme Disease." *Explore!* 18, no. 6 (November). Archived at https://www.betterhealthguy.com/images/stories/PDF/kpu_klinghardt_explore_18-6.pdf.

Goswami, Neela D., Christopher D. Pfeiffer, John R. Horton, Karen Chiswell, Asba Tasneem, and Ephraim L. Tsalik. 2016. "The State of Infectious Diseases Clinical Trials: A Systematic Review of ClinicalTrials.gov." *PLoS One* 8, no. 10 (October): e77086. https://doi.org/10.1371/journal.pone.0077086.

Gupta, Sandeep. Mold Illness (website and online course): https://www.moldillnessmadesimple.com/.

Gukasyan, Natalie, Alan K. Davis, Frederick S. Barrett, Mary P. Cosimano, Nathan D. Sepeda, Matthew W. Johnson, and Roland R. Griffiths. 2022. "Efficacy and Safety of Psilocybin-Assisted Treatment for Major Depressive Disorder: Prospective 12-Month Follow-Up." *Journal of Psychopharmacology* 36, no. 2 (February): 151–158. https://doi.org/10.1177/02698811211073759.

Gustafson, Craig. 2017. "Bruce Lipton, PhD: The Jump from Cell Culture to Consciousness." *Integrative Medicine* (Encinitas) 16, no. 6 (December): 44–50. https://www.ncbi.nlm.nih.gov/pmc/articles/PMC6438088/.

Gutkin, Cal. 2009. "Outliers: Extended Families, Better Health Outcomes: Why Everyone Should Have a Family Doctor." *Canadian Family Physician* 55, no. 7 (July): 768. https://www.cfp.ca/content/cfp/55/7/768.full.pdf.

Heckenlively, Kent, and Judy Mikovits. 2014. *Plague: One Scientist's Intrepid Search for the Truth about Human Retroviruses and Chronic Fatigue Syndrome (ME/CFS), Autism, and Other Diseases.* New York: Skyhorse Publishing.

Hoffman, David. 2003. *Medical Herbalism: The Science and Practice of Herbalism*. Rochester, VT: Healing Arts Press.

Hook, Sarah A., Seonghye Jeon, Sara A. Niesobecki, AmberJean P. Hansen, James I. Meek, Jenna K. H. Bjork, Franny M. Dorr, et al. 2022. "Economic Burden of Reported Lyme Disease in High-Incidence Areas, United States, 2014–2016." *Emerging Infectious Diseases* 28, no. 6 (June): 1170–1179. https://doi.org/10.3201/eid2806.211335.

Hopper, Annie. 2014. *Wired for Healing: Remapping the Brain to Recover from Chronic and Mysterious Illnesses*. Victoria, BC: The Dynamic Neural Retraining System.

Houlihan, Jane, Timothy Kropp, Richard Wiles, Sean Gray, and Chris Campbell. 2005. *Body Burden: The Pollution in Newborns*. Washington, DC: Environmental Working Group. https://www.ewg.org/research/body-burden-pollution-newborns.

Hróbjartsson, Asbjørn, and Peter C. Gøtzsche. 2010. "Placebo Interventions for All Clinical Conditions." *Cochrane Database of Systematic Reviews*, no. 1: CD003974. https://doi.org/10.1002/14651858.CD003974.pub3.

ILADS Working Group. 2014. "Evidence-Based Guidelines for the Management of Lyme Disease." *Expert Review of Anti-Infective Theory* 2, supplement 1 (January): S1–S13. https://doi.org/10.1586/14789072.2.1.S1.

Institute of Medicine. 2011. "Federal Funding of Tick-Borne Diseases." In *Critical Needs and Gaps in Understanding Prevention, Amelioration, and Resolution of Lyme and Other Tick-Borne Diseases: The Short-Term and Long-Terms Outcomes: Workshop Report*. Washington, DC: National Academies Press. https://doi.org/10.17226/13134.

Institute of Medicine and National Research Council. 2009. "Drivers of Zoonotic Diseases." In *Sustaining Global Surveillance and Response to Emerging Zoonotic Diseases*. Gerald T. Keusch, Marguerite Pappaioanou, Mila C. Gonzalez, Kimberly A. Scott, and Peggy Tsai, eds. Washington, DC: National Academies Press. https://doi.org/10.17226/12625.

Janjua Ullah, Hafeez, Munir Akhtar, and Fayyaz Hussain. 2016. "Effects of Sugar, Salt and Distilled Water on White Blood Cells and Platelet Cells." *Journal of Tumor* 4, no. 1: 354–358. https://doi.org/10.17554/j.issn.1819-6187.2016.04.73.

Johnson, Lorraine. 2019. *2019 Chart Book: MyLymeData Registry.* LymeDisease.org. https://www.lymedisease.org/2019-mylymedata-highlights.pdf.

Kabat-Zinn, Jon. 2013. *Full Catastrophe Living: Using the Wisdom of Your Body and Mind to Face Stress, Pain, and Illness.* Revised ed. New York: Bantam.

Laukkanen, Tanjaniina, Hassan Khan, Francesco Zaccardi, and Jari A. Laukkanen. 2015. "Association between Sauna Bathing and Fatal Cardiovascular and All-Cause Mortality Events." *JAMA Internal Medicine* 175, no. 4 (April): 542–548. https://doi.org/10.1001/jamainternmed.2014.8187.

Levitt, B. Blake. 1995. *Electromagnetic Fields: A Consumer's Guide to the Issues and How to Protect Ourselves.* San Diego: Harcourt Brace.

Liebert, Matthew D., Johanna M. Jarcho, Steve Berman, Bruce D. Naliboff, Brandall Y. Suyenobu, Mark Mandelkern, and Emeran A. Mayer. 2004. "The Neural Correlates of Placebo Effects: A Disruption Account." *NeuroImage* 22, no. 1 (May): 447–455. https://doi.org/10.1016/j.neuroimage.2004.01.037.

Liegner, Kenneth B. 2019. "Disulfiram (Tetrathylthiuram Disulfide) in the Treatment of Lyme Disease and Babesiosis: Report of Experience in Three Cases." *Antibiotics* 8, no. 2 (June): 72. https://doi.org/10.3390/antibiotics8020072.

Light, Kathleen C., Karen M. Grewen, and Janet A. Amico. 2005. "More Frequent Partner Hugs and Higher Oxytocin Levels Are Linked to Lower Blood Pressure and Heart Rate in Premenopausal Women." *Biological Psychology* 69, no. 1 (April): 5–21. https://doi.org/10.1016/j.biopsycho.2004.11.002.

Lin, Steven. 2018. *The Dental Diet: The Surprising Link between Your Teeth, Real Food, and Life-Changing Natural Health*. Carlsbad, CA: Hay House.

Lipton, Bruce H. 2005. *The Biology of Belief: Unleashing the Power of Consciousness, Matter & Miracles*. Carlsbad, CA: Hay House.

Locey, Kenneth J., and Jay T. Lennon. 2016. "Scaling Laws Predict Global Microbial Diversity." *PNAS* 113, no. 21 (May): 5970–5975. https://doi.org/10.1073/pnas.1521291113.

Loftfield, Erikka, Joseph A. Rothwell, Rashmi Sinha, Pekka Keski-Rahkonen, Nivonirina Robinot, Demetrius Albanes, Stephanie J. Weinstein, et al. 2020. "Prospective Investigation of Serum Metabolites, Coffee Drinking, Liver Cancer Incidence, and Liver Disease Mortality." *Journal of the National Cancer Institute* 112, no. 3 (March): 286–294. https://doi.org/10.1093/jnci/djz122.

Lyme Disease Wonk. 2019. "Prevalence of Lyme Disease Is a Big and Growing Problem—Let's Look at the Numbers." *MyLymeData Viz Blog*. January 3, 2019. https://www.lymedisease.org/mylymedata-lyme-disease-prevalence/.

Manné, Joy. 2009. *Family Constellations: A Practical Guide to Uncovering the Origins of Family Conflict*. Berkeley: North Atlantic Books.

Marshall, Vincent. 1988. "Multiple Sclerosis Is a Chronic Central Nervous System Infection by a Spirochetal Agent." *Medical Hypotheses* 25, no. 2 (February): 89–92. https://doi.org/10.1016/0306-9877(88)90023-0.

Martinez, Marisol. 2022. "Psilocybin Treatment for Major Depression Effective for Up to a Year for Most Patients, Study Shows." Hub, John Hopkins University. February 16, 2022. https://hub.jhu.edu/2022/02/16/psilocybin-relieves-depression-for-up-to-a-year/.

Maté, Gabor. 2003. *When the Body Says No: Understanding the Stress-Disease Connection*. Hoboken, NJ: Wiley.

McFadzean, Nicola. 2010. *The Lyme Diet: Nutritional Strategies for Healing from Lyme Disease*. South Lake Tahoe, CA: BioMed Publishing Group.

McMakin, Carolyn. 2017. *The Resonance Effect: How Frequency Specific Microcurrent Is Changing Medicine*. Berkeley, CA: North Atlantic Books.

Meinig, George E. 2008. *Root Canal Cover-Up*. Lemon Grove, CA: Price-Pottenger Nutrition Foundation.

Mercola, Joseph. 2022. "Are EMFs—Electromagnetic Fields—Hazardous to Our Health?" Mercola.com, January 21, 2008. Accessed August 20, 2022. Archived at https://www.bibliotecapleyades.net/scalar_tech/esp_scalartech_cellphonesmicrowave11.htm.

Middelveen, Marianne J., Jennie Burke, Eva Sapi, Cheryl Bandoski, Katherine R. Filush, Yean Wang, Agustin Franco, et al. 2014. "Culture and Identification of *Borrelia* Spirochetes in Human Vaginal and Seminal Secretions." *F1000Research* 3, no. 309 (December). https://doi.org/10.12688/f1000research.5778.3.

Moritz, Andreas. 1998. *The Amazing Liver and Gallbladder Flush: A Powerful Do-It-Yourself Approach to Optimize Your Health and Well-Being...and Much More!* Ener-Chi Wellness Press.

Moseley, J. Bruce, Kimberly O'Malley, Nancy J. Petersen, Terri J. Menke, Baruch A. Brody, David H. Kuykendall, John C. Hollingsworth, Carol M. Ashton, and Nelda P. Wray. 2002. "A Controlled Trial of Arthroscopic Surgery for Osteoarthritis of the Knee." *New England Journal of Medicine* 347, no. 2 (July): 81–88. https://doi.org/10.1056/NEJMoa013259.

Naiman, Rubin. 2014. *Hush: A Book of Bedtime Contemplations*. Tucson: New Moon Media.

NASA. 2020. "Effects of Isolation and Confinement on Hippocampal Volume and Visuo-Spatial Memory." NASA Life Sciences Portal: Record Viewer. Last updated June 10, 2020. https://lsda.jsc.nasa.gov/Experiment/exper/13775.

Nathan, Neil. 2018. *Toxic: Heal Your Body from Mold Toxicity, Lyme Disease, Multiple Chemical Sensitivities, and Chronic Environmental Illness*. Las Vegas: Victory Belt Publishing.

———. 2022. *Energetic Diagnosis: Groundbreaking Thesis on Diagnosing Disease and Chronic Illness*. Las Vegas: Victory Belt Publishing.

Nestor, James. 2020. *Breath: The New Science of a Lost Art*. New York: Riverhead Books.

Newby, Kris. 2019. *Bitten: The Secret History of Lyme Disease and Biological Weapons*. New York: Harper Wave.

Northrup, Christiane. 2018. *Dodging Energy Vampires: An Empath's Guide to Evading Relationships That Drain You and Restoring Your Health and Power*. Carlsbad, CA: Hay House.

Oschman, James L., Gaétan Chevalier, and Richard Brown. 2015. "The Effects of Grounding (Earthing) on Inflammation, the Immune Response, Wound Healing, and Prevention and Treatment of Chronic Inflammatory and Autoimmune Diseases." *Journal of Inflammation Research* 2015, no. 8 (March): 83–96. https://doi.org/10.2147/JIR.S69656.

Pall, Martin L. 2018. "Wi-Fi Is an Important Threat to Human Health." *Environmental Research* 164 (July): 405–416. https://doi.org/10.1016/j.envres.2018.01.035.

Pert, Candace B. 1997. *Molecules of Emotion: The Science behind Mind-Body Medicine*. New York: Scribner.

Petrison, Lisa, and Erik Johnson. 2015. *A Beginner's Guide to Mold Avoidance: Techniques Used by Thousands of Chronic Multisystem Illness Sufferers to Improve Their Health*. Paradigm Change/Lisa Petrison and Erik Johnson.

Pfeiffer, Mary Beth. 2018. *Lyme: The First Epidemic of Climate Change*. Washington, DC: Island Press.

Phillips, Steven, and Dana Parish. 2020. *Chronic: The Hidden Cause of the Autoimmune Epidemic and How to Get Healthy Again*. Boston: Houghton Mifflin Harcourt.

Pineault, Nicolas. 2019. *The Non-Tinfoil Guide to EMFs: How to Fix Our Stupid Use of Technology*. N&G Media.

Plevin, Julia. 2019. *Healing Magic of Forest Bathing: Finding Calm, Creativity, and Connection in the Natural World*. Berkeley, CA: Ten Speed Press.

Ragozzino, Claire. 2020. *Living Ayurveda: Nourishing Body and Mind through Seasonal Recipes, Rituals, and Yoga*. Boulder, CO: Roost Books.

Ramesh, Geeta, Lenay Santana-Gould, Fiona M. Inglis, John D. England, and Maria T. Philip. 2013. "The Lyme Disease Spirochete *Borrelia burgdorferi* Induces Inflammation and Apoptosis in Cells from Dorsal Root Ganglia." *Journal of Neuroinflammation* 10, no. 88: 865. https://doi.org/10.1186/1742-2094-10-88.

Ramirez, Francisco E., Albert Sanchez, and Aki T. Pirskanen. 2021. "Hydrothermotherapy in Prevention and Treatment of Mild to Moderate Cases of COVID-19." *Medical Hypotheses* 146, no. 110363 (January). https://doi.org/10.1016/j.mehy.2020.110363.

Raxlen, Bernard. 2019. *Lyme Disease: Medical Myopia and the Hidden Global Pandemic*. London: Hammersmith Health Books.

Reuben, Suzanne H. 2010. *Reducing Environmental Cancer Risk: What We Can Do Now*. U.S. Department of Health and Human Services. April 2010. https://deainfo.nci.nih.gov/advisory/pcp/annualreports/pcp08-09rpt/pcp_report_08-09_508.pdf.

Rosenberg, Stanley. 2017. *Accessing the Healing Power of the Vagus Nerve: Self-Help Exercises for Anxiety, Depression, Trauma, and Autism*. Berkeley, CA: North Atlantic Books.

Rothbaum, Barbara Olasov. 1997. "A Controlled Study of Eye Movement Desensitization and Reprocessing in the Treatment of Posttraumatic Stress Disordered Sexual Assault Victims." *Bulletin of the Menninger Clinic* 61, no. 3 (Summer): 317–334. https://pubmed.ncbi.nlm.nih.gov/9260344/.

Schafer, Kristin S., Margaret Reeves, Skip Spitzer, and Susan E. Kegley. 2004. *Chemical Trespass: Pesticides in Our Bodies and Corporate Accountability*. San Francisco: Pesticide Action Network North America (PANNA). https://www.panna.org/sites/default/files/ChemTres2004Eng.pdf.

Shallenberger, Frank. 2017. *The Ozone Miracle: How You Can Harness the Power of Oxygen to Keep You and Your Family Healthy.* Self-published.

Shan, Jinyu, Ying Jia, Louis Teulières, Faizal Patel, and Martha R. J. Clokie. 2021. "Targeting Multicopy Prophage Genes for the Increased Detection of *Borrelia burgdorferi* Sensu Lato (s.l.), the Causative Agents of Lyme Disease, in Blood." *Frontiers in Microbiology* 12, no. 651217 (March). https://doi.org/10.3389/fmicb.2021.651217.

Shapiro, Francine. 2014. "The Role of Eye Movement Desensitization and Reprocessing (EMDR) Therapy in Medicine: Addressing the Psychological and Physical Symptoms Stemming from Adverse Life Experiences." *The Permanente Journal* 18, no. 1 (Winter): 71–77. https://doi.org/10.7812/TPP/13-098.

Shoemaker, Ritchie C. 2005. *Mold Warriors: Fighting Americas Hidden Health Threat.* Louisville, KY: Gateway Press.

Sonenshine, Daniel E., and Kevin R. Macaluso. 2017. "Microbial Invasion vs. Tick Immune Regulation." *Frontiers in Cellular and Infection Microbiology* 7, no. 390 (September). https://doi.org/10.3389/fcimb.2017.00390.

Stapleton, P., J. Dispenza, S. McGill, D. Sabot, M. Peach, and D. Raynor. 2020. "Large Effects of Brief Meditation Intervention on EEG Spectra in Meditation Novices." *IBRO Reports* 9 (December): 290–301. https://doi.org/10.1016/j.ibror.2020.10.006.

Stechenberg, Barbara W. 1988. "Lyme Disease: The Latest Great Imitator." *The Pediatric Infectious Disease Journal* 7, no. 6 (June): 402–409. https://doi.org/10.1097/00006454-198806000-00007.

Stricker, Raphael B., and Lorraine Johnson. 2010. "Lyme Disease Diagnosis and Treatment: Lessons from the AIDS Epidemic." *Minerva Medica* 101, no. 6 (December): 419–425. https://www.minervamedica.it/index2.t?show=R10Y2010N06A0419.

Stricker, Raphael B., and Melissa C. Fesler. 2018. "Chronic Lyme Disease: A Working Case Definition." *American Journal of Infectious Diseases* 14, no. 1: 1–44. https://doi.org/10.3844/ajidsp.2018.1.44.

Stricker, Raphael B., Joseph Burrascano, and Edward Winger. 2002. "Longterm Decrease in the CD57 Lymphocyte Subset in a Patient with Chronic Lyme Disease." *Annals of Agricultural and Environmental Medicine* 9, no. 1 (February): 111–113. https://www.anapsid.org/cnd/files/strickercd57.pdf.

Tennant, Jerry L. 2014. *Healing Is Voltage: The Handbook.* 3rd ed. Self-published.

Tickell, Joshua, and Rebecca Harrell Tickell, directors. 2019. *The Earthing Movie: The Remarkable Science of Grounding.* Big Picture Ranch. https://www.youtube.com/watch?v=44ddtRoXDVU.

Tilburt, Jon C., Ezekiel J. Emanuel, Ted J. Kaptchuk, Farr A. Curlin, and Franklin G. Miller. 2008. "Prescribing 'Placebo Treatments': Results of National Survey of US Internists and Rheumatologists." *BJM* 337, no. a1938. https://doi.org/10.1136/bmj.a1938.

van der Kolk, Bessel. 2014. *The Body Keeps the Score: Brain, Mind, and Body in the Healing of Trauma.* New York: Penguin.

Van Such, Monica, Robert Lohr, Thomas Beckman, James M. Naessens. 2017. "Extent of Diagnostic Agreement Among Medical Referrals." *Journal of Evaluation in Clinical Practice* 23, no. 4 (August): 870–874. https://doi.org/10.1111/jep.12747.

Wahls, Terry, and Eve Adamson. 2014. *The Wahls Protocol: A Radical New Way to Treat All Chronic Autoimmune Conditions Using Paleo Principles.* Revised ed. New York: Avery.

Walker, Matthew. 2017. *Why We Sleep: Unlocking the Power of Sleep and Dreams.* New York: Scribner.

Walter, Katherine S., Giovanna Carpi, Adalgisa Caccone, and Maria A. Diuk-Wasser. 2017. "Genomic Insights into the Ancient Spread of Lyme Disease across North America." *Nature Ecology & Evolution* 1 (October): 1569–1576. https://doi.org/10.1038/s41559-017-0282-8.

Wartolowska, Karolina, Andrew Judge, Sally Hopewell, Gary S. Collins, Benjamin J.F. Dean, Ines Rombach, David Brindley, Julian Savulescu, David J. Beard, and Andrew J. Carr. 2014. "Use of Placebo Controls in the Evaluation of Surgery: Systematic Review." *BMJ* 348, no. g3253. https://doi.org/10.1136/bmj.g3253.

Wass, Tara, and Kaia Gallagher. 2008. "Evaluation of Heavy Metals Levels in Relation to Ionic Foot Bath Sessions with the Ioncleanse®." Center for Research Strategies. June 30, 2008. http://www.ahrfoundation.net/dlfiles/study_results.pdf.

Weber, Hans Michael, Yasaman Zandi Mehran, Armin Orthaber, Hadi Hosseini Saadat, Robert Weber, and Matthias Wojcik. 2020. "Successful Reduction of SARS-CoV-2 Viral Load by Photodynamic Therapy (PDT) Verified by QPCR – A Novel Approach in Treating Patients in Early Infection Stages." *Medical & Clinical Research* 5, no. 11: 311–325. https://www.medclinrese.org/open-access/successful-reduction-of-sarscov2-viral-load-by-photodynamic-therapy-pdt-verified-by-qpcra-novel-approach-in-treating-pat.pdf.

Wilker, S., A. Pfeiffer, S. Kolassa, T. Elbert, B. Lingenfelder, E. Ovuga, A. Papassotiropoulos, D. de Quervain, and I.-T. Kolassa. 2014. "The Role of *FKBP5* Genotype in Moderating Long-Term Effectiveness of Exposure-Based Psychotherapy for Posttraumatic Stress Disorder." *Translational Psychiatry* 4, no. e403. https://doi.org/10.1038/tp.2014.49.

Williams, Louisa L. 2011. *Radical Medicine: Cutting-Edge Natural Therapies That Treat the Root Causes of Disease.* Rochester, VT: Healing Arts Press.

Williamson, Elizabeth, Samuel Driver, and Karen Baxter, eds. 2009. *Stockley's Herbal Medicines Interactions.* London/Grayslake, IL: Pharmaceutical Press. https://www.stonybrookmedicine.edu/sites/default/files/herbal_medicines_interactions-1.pdf.

Wilson, Gemma et al. 2018. "The Use of Eye-Movement Desensitization Reprocessing (EMDR) Therapy in Treating Post-Traumatic Stress Disorder—A Systematic Narrative Review." *Frontiers in Psychology* 9, no. 923 (June). https://doi.org/10.3389%2Ffpsyg.2018.00923.

Wilson, S. A., L. A. Becker, and R. H. Tinker. 1995. "Eye Movement Desensitization and Reprocessing (EMDR) Treatment for Psychologically Traumatized Individuals." *Journal of Consulting and Clinical Psychology* 63, no. 6: 928–937. https://doi.org/10.1037/0022-006X.63.6.928.

———. 1997. "Fifteen-Month Follow-Up of Eye Movement Desensitization and Reprocessing (EMDR) Treatment for Posttraumatic Stress Disorder and Psychological Trauma." *Journal of Consulting and Clinical Psychology*, 65, no. 6: 1047–1056. https://doi.org/10.1037/0022-006X.65.6.1047.

Wolynn, Mark. 2016. *It Didn't Start with You: How Inherited Family Trauma Shapes Who We Are and How to End the Cycle.* New York: Penguin Life.

Woitzel, Ingo. Private medical practice in Germany: https://dr-woitzel.de/.

Young, Robert O., and Shelly Redford Young. 2002. *The pH Miracle: Balance Your Diet, Reclaim Your Health.* New York: Warner Books.

Zhang, Xinzhi, Martin I. Meltzer, César A. Peña, Annette B. Hopkins, Lane Wroth, and Alan D. Fix. 2006. "Economic Impact of Lyme Disease." *Emerging Infectious Diseases* 12, no. 4 (April): 653–660. https://doi.org/10.3201/eid1204.050602.

Zhang, Xue-Chao, Zhang-Nv Yang, Bo Lu, Xiao-Fang Ma, Chuan-Xi Zhang, and Hai-Jun Xu. 2014. "The Composition and Transmission of Microbiome in Hard Tick, *Ixodes persulcatus*, during Blood Meal." *Tick and Tick-Borne Diseases* 5, no. 6 (October): 964–870. https://doi.org/10.1016/j.ttbdis.2014.07.009.

Zimmer, Carl. 2000. *Parasite Rex: Inside the Bizarre World of Nature's Most Dangerous Creatures.* New York: Atria Books.

GLOSSARY

Bay Area Lyme Foundation: a national organization committed to making Lyme Disease easy to diagnose and simple to cure.

Borrelia burgdorferi: a bacterial species of the spirochete class in the genus *Borrelia* and is the main causative agent of Lyme Disease in humans.

C4A: blood level of C4 proteins, which play a role in how the immune system functions. When C4A is high, it means the immune system is working hard to clear pathogens and toxins.

CD57: the amount of positive NK cells. The lower the amount of CD57 natural killer cells in the body, the more chronic the Lyme Disease is, and the higher the amount, the closer a person is to remission.

Chronic Inflammatory Response Syndrome (CIRS): a complex illness characterized by exposure to biotoxins and ongoing inflammation in the body affecting multiple organs and systems.

Chrysanthemum: a flower that deters fleas and ticks from the backyard or surroundings. Its oil is used in bug sprays and other insect repellents.

Cytokines: a category of small proteins important in cell signaling made by various types of white blood cells to turn on the immune system to attack invaders. Although these proteins play a vital role for normal immune function, when produced in excess in the context of Lyme Disease, they produce many unwanted symptoms.

DEET: the active ingredient in many insect repellent products. When applied, it protects by preventing mosquitoes or other insects from landing on skin or clothing.

DMSA: substance that chelates mercury and lead which is used in a test to show their respective levels in the body.

EAV device: a noninvasive assessment tool that can help to evaluate health issues through measuring the body's energy using acupuncture points on the skin.

EDTA: substance that chelates several heavy metals which is used to show their respective levels in the body.

Enzyme-linked immunosorbent assay (ELISA): a test for detecting and quantifying substances such as peptides, proteins, antibodies, and hormones. In the case of Lyme, it detects antibodies to *B. burgdorferi*.

Epstein Barr Virus (EBV): known as human herpesvirus 4, is a member of the herpes virus family and is one of the most common human viruses. In the case of chronic Lyme, EBV can become active from a previously dormant or latent state.

Erythema migrans: a rash that frequently appears as a tell-tale symptom of Lyme Disease at the location of the insect bite. It's typically a circular red area appearing in the form of a bull's-eye pattern.

flagellum: a tail-like structure that enables the spirochete to move throughout the body.

Global Lyme Alliance: an organization dedicated to advancing Lyme Disease research and improving the quality of life of those living with Lyme through research, education, awareness, and other programs.

Infectious Diseases Society of America (IDSA): a medical association that does not recognize the persistence of the bacteria in chronic Lyme and instead considers chronic Lyme "Post-Lyme Disease Syndrome."

International Lyme and Associated Diseases Society (ILADS): a nonprofit, international, multidisciplinary medical society, committed to the diagnosis and appropriate treatment of Lyme and its associated coinfections. ILADS recognizes chronic Lyme as a serious, challenging condition that requires a specialized treatment approach and promotes its awareness in the greater medical community and public at large.

Lyme-literate doctor (LLMD): a physician who is familiar with the symptoms that may indicate Lyme Disease infection at various stages of the disease, as well as potential coinfections and other complexities and has the specific knowledge and experience to treat the disease.

National Institutes of Health (NIH): the primary agency of the US government responsible for biomedical and public health research.

photosensitizer: molecules that absorb light and transfer its energy into another nearby molecule.

transcutaneous electrical nerve stimulation (TENS): a device that sends electrical pulses through the skin using a mild electrical current.

Western blot: a widely used analytical technique in molecular biology and immunogenetics to detect specific proteins in a sample of tissue homogenate or extract.

ABOUT THE AUTHOR

I grew up on the west coast of Canada in beautiful British Columbia. I started my career as an entrepreneur in e-commerce after studying systems engineering. I built one of the major online payment companies in Mexico. Then after almost a decade of entrepreneurship, I became sick and realized that I needed to drastically change my lifestyle and perspective. After I understood that the conventional medical community couldn't help me, I dropped everything and dedicated all my energy to healing. Now on the other side of the illness, I feel extremely humbled with a responsibility to give back to the community as so many people helped me on my own journey. I wrote this book because I wanted to put what I learned on my own journey to use and share the information with others.

I'm grateful for all the healers and beautiful souls whom I encountered, ranging from shamans, naturopaths, acupuncturists, homeopathic doctors, PhD students, biological dentists, to trauma healers and multiple other experts who helped me along the way. Today, I live my life with the practices I learned over the last few years to heal from Lyme and maintain an openness to continued learning on health and wellness topics. I try to grow my own food and ensure that I live in a clean environment. I'm more conscious of how my actions impact the earth and nurture a connection to my natural environment. At the same time, I try not to take myself too seriously and always make time for play and movement. I strive to surround myself with a community that I love and that loves me back and to always feel aligned with where I spend my energy.

www.ingramcontent.com/pod-product-compliance
Lightning Source LLC
Chambersburg PA
CBHW020458030426
42337CB00011B/149